i

Intermittent Fasting Guide: Super-Charged Results for Energy, Health, and Weight Loss

Intermittent Fasting Guide: Super-Charged Results for Energy, Health, and Weight Loss

Includes 30 Recipes and an
Intermittent Fasting Meal Plan

Kyle Faber

Intermittent Fasting Guide: Super-Charged Results for Energy, Health, and Weight Loss

Heal Your Body Through a Return to Healthy Eating Patterns

Published by CAC Publishing LLC.

ISBN 978-1-948489-97-3 paperback

ISBN 978-1-948489-96-6 eBook

This book is not intended for the purpose of providing medical advice.

All information, content, and material of this book is for informational purposes only and is not intended to serve as a substitute for the consultation, diagnosis, and/or medical treatment of a qualified physician or healthcare provider. The reader should always consult his or her healthcare provider to determine the appropriateness of the information for his or her own situation or if he or she has any questions regarding a medical condition or treatment plan.

Contents

Chapter 1: Why Intermittent Fasting?

The Human Inheritance

How we eat has a direct impact on how we think, how we feel, how long we live, and how we influence our progeny. The bulk of this book is intended to unravel why we eat the way we do, why we really should change that to eat in a way that helps us reach our full potential – and how intermittent fasting can help us do that.

Before we can really talk about intermittent fasting, we need to begin with two premises. First, our human physiology is the aggregate result of the environments around us. Those environments include the physical environment, the elements and nature; the psychological environment, our thoughts and feelings; and the intangible environment both within and surrounding us. Second, we are the culminative result of the generations that have come before. The human mind, body, and spirit are like an organic blockchain (to borrow a term from a technology). We have been impacted by and are the result of what our predecessors did as far back as the first single-celled organisms. Conversely, each thing we do now will have an impact on the generations to come.

So, let's start with a little history and look at how we evolved to get to where we are now.

Human beings weren't always the dominant species on the planet, and our ancestors were not always at the top of the food chain. Everything we now take for granted, from buildings that scrape the sky, to the planes that fly across it, to writing and computers and all the technological and scientific advances of mankind, are all things that have happened in the last 10,000 years. That may seem like a long time because our average individual lifespan is a mere 0.007% of that, but 10,000 years is a drop in the bucket compared to the 6 million years it has been since humans were arboreal, or the 20 million years that it took human beings to stand upright as we do now.

As human beings evolved, so did their eating habits. At some distant point in our common history, our ancestors began to change the way they consumed their nutritional requirements. Whether by necessity or opportunity, mankind shifted from being scavengers to becoming hunter-gatherers. They stopped needing to raid the carcasses of larger prey after the lions and hyenas had had their fill.

Then, as our ancestors developed tools and fire, their eating habits changed even more, and human beings were catapulted to the top of the food chain. Once they began cooking food, early man was able to eat less, because more was nutritionally available from each portion of food, and because cooked food needed less digestive processing, that energy was redirected to cognitive development.

It turns out that we owe much of our intelligence to man's mastery of fire and becoming able to cook our food! As our brains grew, we no longer needed to scavenge the food that other animals, like lions, hunted. We started making tools, and extended our abilities further using external objects. Not only did we diversify our sources of energy – fruits, seeds, berries, and whatever we could gather in the fields and forest – but we could now organize and hunt prey of our own. By the time the Paleolithic age rolled around, we had graduated to being hunter-gatherers, hunting prey and gathering food. As the quality of our food increased, mortality rates decreased, and human populations increased.

Hunting and gathering also played into a new pattern that was forming – our ancestors began to travel. They would harvest all they could from wherever they were, and when there was nothing left to forage, they would pack up and leave in search of the next area that would offer them bounty. A nomadic strain was added to our genes, becoming another part of our heritage. Small groups would forage a location, exhaust all it had to offer, and then move on to the next spot. Two key developments happened in this line of humans: first, their eating patterns became entrenched in human biology, and, second, they started forming organized groups.

The bulk of the nutrition consumed by our biological ancestors came from meat they hunted, supplemented by the seeds, fruits, grains, and roots they found in the areas they settled in. For a million years, the majority of their energy needs was supplied by prey – meat. What they ate, when they ate, and how much they ate helped shape human physiology of eating and digestion, and the distribution and use of energy and nutrients in the human body all the way into the modern era.

Most importantly, our ancestors experienced feast or famine as the overriding pattern of the day. With no refrigeration or no other technologies to stop the decay of meat after slaughter, these hunter-gatherers had two options. They could either eat everything or let it rot. So they would eat everything and share their food with the whole community. Whenever there was meat from prey, they feasted. That would be a high protein meal with a high fat content. When there was no prey to provide that meat, they had little to nothing to eat.

Over time, the human body of our ancestors adapted. Their metabolic processes adapted, developing an efficient way to handle cycles of feast and famine. The human body developed a more robust fuel tank system. Of all the food that they ate, which was large in quantity during times of abundance, some was converted to glycogen for liver and muscle storage, and the rest was converted into fat and distributed over the body. It is an efficient system. Instead of having a single storage location, the human body uses the surface layer under the skin, an expandable and contractible organ, to store the fat as it became available. The human body also kept some readily available energy in the form of glycogen in the liver and muscles. That could be easily converted to fuel when needed. The rest of the stored energy would need to go through a specific metabolic cycle to convert the stored fat back into usable energy.

On the day after a feast, the group wouldn't need to hunt, and they would be full and satiated. The body would divert its energy resources from the brain and the limbs to the digestive system to aid the process of digesting all that food and the distribution of those nutrients and fats. This would be a basically lazy day. If they needed something else to sustain them, they still had things like fruits and seeds to eat.

During those first hours, energy in the form of glycogen would supply their basic energy needs, from keeping their brain functional to having energy available for defense if needed. However, that glycogen source was not designed to last very long. Once it was depleted, the body would switch to using the fat stored subcutaneously. At that point, the satiated and related feelings from the feast would dissipate as the byproducts of the alternate fat-burning metabolic processes would begin to fuel their brains – and that would be like a shot of caffeine.

All this meant that an early hunter-gatherer had two tools that allowed him to rapidly climb to the top of the food chain. First, he had a significant amount of energy to draw from – more than just the glycogen stores that fed him during the first day after the feast. He had pure concentrated energy in the form of fat that could be converted back into energy to power his muscles. A byproduct of that conversion, ketones, could power his brain, giving his brain an extra boost. The combined effect of increasing muscular power (resulting in speed and endurance) and a more robust brain allowed early man to outsmart his prey and have the energy to outrun his prey. While man was not faster than most of the prey he targeted, he was certainly smarter and could keep going even after the animal became incapacitated from exhaustion.

That is our human legacy. That is the way our bodies and brains have evolved. We have the potential to power our brains and our intelligence, and the power to have strong and resilient bodies – if we manage our energy profiles correctly to take advantage of that legacy.

But our human history didn't end there. Our ancestors continued to develop. They learned the benefits of living in larger groups, and started to learn how to farm. Farming allowed them to stay in one place longer because they no longer had to migrate when the resources of an area were exhausted. Agriculture developed to include the organized planting and harvesting of fruits, vegetables, and grains, as well as the raising of various types of livestock. This caused major shifts in the eating habits and energy profiles that had proved so beneficial to humankind up to that point.

Organized farming, and the subsequent expansion of bartering and monetary stores of value, saw the advance of specialization. Specialization allowed a goat herder to focus on his goats while the zucchini farmer could specialize in zucchinis. Specialization resulted in better rates of food production and increased value. Small villages grew into large cities and entire civilizations were born to facilitate trade. This also meant that there were all kinds of people selling all kinds of things, just as it is today, making a broader range of food choices available to more people more of the time. This, above all, has had the greatest impact on human eating habits and energy profiles.

But not all more recent developments in human eating patterns result in improved health and energy. Take, for example, the prevalence of cow's milk in the diets of people around the world. The human gastrointestinal process didn't develop to process cow's milk. Our ancient ancestors didn't stop to take the milk of other species; they didn't stop to milk a buffalo, ox, or cow. Milk didn't become a regular part of the human diet until cattle farmers began to harvest and sell everything they could from a cow, from the skin as leather, to crushed bones as fertilizer, and to milk as a beverage. This was so successful that milk, no longer an ancillary industry to the meat, became an entirely mature industry of its own. Unfortunately, no matter how much we are convinced that milk is good for us, milk is just not something that human bodies can break down and extract full benefit from. Even the calcium from milk is not fully bioavailable. One in five children in the United States have milk allergies, and that's the ones we know about. There are many more, probably as many as three in five, that have minor allergies that go unreported. Human beings didn't evolve to drink milk the milk of other species, and yet we do.

Intermittent fasting is normal

Despite changes to human eating habits over more recent history, we need to remember that human physiology originally developed under conditions that favored the consumption of certain foods and where eating was not a daily occurrence. Human beings evolved to eat a large quantity of food, store it, and then survive on that stored energy for a few days. Once that store was depleted, humans would hunt and forage for more food. It's not just about how much we ate, it's also about how often and when we ate.

This brings us to the topic of our book, intermittent fasting. At its most basic, intermittent fasting is about when you eat, not so much about what you eat.

"Intermittent fasting" falsely conjures up an impression of difficulty and discomfort, and triggers an aversion to what is actually a natural thing for humans. We tend to see fasting as synonymous with starving, but it is not. Fasting and starving have very different clinical definitions. Fasting is when you stop using the food that you have eaten most recently as the source of energy, whereas starvation occurs when your body no longer has any stores of fat left to convert to energy and begins to convert muscle mass – in other words, the body starts attacking living tissue – to fuel essential systems. Most of us, even if we haven't eaten for a week, are nowhere near starving.

Re-evaluating our eating habits

When we begin to reconsider how we function, including the way we eat, we need to take into account three areas. The first is the machinery of the body with all its structures, tissues, and processes. The second is our brain, the seat of control and consciousness. The brain controls appetite, homeostasis, and even sleep cycles. Third is the environment around us. Not just the natural world or the air and water that sustains us, the environment is also about what we are influenced to do – the actions we mimic, the trends we follow, the culture we are a part of. Even the prevailing political climate is part of the environment that influences our health and well-being. So, in looking at intermittent fasting, we'll need to look at it from the physical and physiological standpoint, the mental standpoint, and the cultural or environmental perspective.

One of the recurring themes you'll find in this book are the role of habits in eating and fasting. Our eating habits can be like slowly accumulating toxins in more than one way. (And, as you'll see, intermittent fasting can help clear that up.)

Let me illustrate this point. If you eat enough of something toxic all at once, you will experience observable repercussions. But if you take the same thing over a long period, and in small enough quantities, you will find that the amounts you ingest that don't exceed the threshold will accumulate instead and have a long-lasting effect on our system which only becomes apparent much later. This is true of arsenic. And it is true of drinking mercury in water.

If arsenic, which is one of the most toxic and lethal substances known to man, can accumulate in the body long before it kills you, then you need to realize that the issue of habit – something that you do repeatedly, and which applies equally to what you eat – can have a significant impact on your life over time.

Human beings are creatures of habit. Once we start a habit it's hard to let go of our personal habits. There are also powerful societal habits, things we do just because that is what everyone around us does. Societal habits can include what we eat, where and when we eat it. Food habits can be based on cultural aspects of food that no longer make sense anymore for changing energy profiles and circumstances.

For example, the Inuit tribes of North America have always hunted whales as part of their diet. Two of the most prized sections of the whale are its skin and blubber, the fat just below the skin. The meat is edible, of course, and is used widely in dishes and recipes. The fat is enjoyed and accepted because it provides a huge amount of energy, fueling the Inuit's metabolism and layering their bodies with the fat necessary to battle the frigid temperatures of the Arctic. However, if an Inuit moves to more temperate latitude along the equator, he couldn't possibly continue eating a diet rich in whale blubber and would find himself battling an old habit that would be trying to override his appetite for something different and more appropriate to eat.

Eating habits and three meals a day

Habits can become established mindsets and biases that aren't supported by real understanding. One such habit is the common belief in the need to eat three square meals a day. There is nothing in our genetic makeup that requires us to eat three meals at predetermined times regardless of our lifestyle. Why would one person who works with heavy physical exertion, lifting large boxes, eat the same amount and on the same schedule as the man who sits at a desk all day watching camera monitors? Their energy requirements and overall profiles are obviously very different. There is a lot more energy expended by the delivery guy doing physical carrying and pushing than there is by a building security specialist at his desk monitoring camera feeds. One could burn 3,000 calories a day, while the other burns just 1,000. Why would it make sense that they both eat a 1,200 calorie lunch? It doesn't. The strenuously active person needs to consume significantly more calories, three times more to be exact.

Eat *what* you need *when* you need it

Each of us has a different energy profile, so it only makes sense that we should all have different consumption patterns. These consumption patterns include optimal timing and the calories required. In intermittent fasting programs, you don't need to worry too much about calories, but your goal should be to find your optimal schedule and frequency of meals. Later, we'll talk about different eating schedules and how to better understand what your appetite is telling you to eat.

Intermittent fasting is not something you will need to follow strictly for the rest of your life. You should practice it until it becomes a habit or a lifestyle. Once you get to that point, eating what you need, when you need it, will be as normal as brushing your teeth. Of course, you can always go back to a period of scheduled intermittent fasting when you want to get your systems back on track.

Although your basic practice of intermittent fasting will be to eat within certain "windows" of time, eating with less frequency, this program also suggests that you need to be eating the right foods. However, it doesn't dictate what those foods are. No one can tell you what the "right" food to eat should be. Only your own body can tell you that, and that is what you want to learn to listen to. The key here is to listen to your own appetite, and then go with it.

Although intermittent fasting is fundamentally about when you eat rather than about what you eat, if you also pay attention to what you eat, you can supercharge your systems – both the gastrointestinal and metabolic systems and their processes – into an even more finely tuned engine with a more beneficial energy profile.

During induction week, there will be a few things that you can do to help your body be better able to tell you exactly what it needs. Then, you will be able to provide your body with exactly the nutrients it is looking for without consuming unnecessary calories.

Appetite Alerts and Cravings

This brings me to the next point of taste and appetite. Your body is a highly complex organism with multiple systems interacting with each other. When you go about your daily routine, the tasks you do cause wear and tear on your systems. It's like a car. You have engine oil in the crankcase to keep the bearings and moving parts lubricated, but once in a while oil levels get too low, and a little light illuminates on the dashboard to tell you that you that the car is low on oil. Then, you need to change the oil or top it up – or, eventually, the car will develop bigger problems.

In the same way, there are many different substances, such as water, that your body needs to perform a broad variety of interactions and processes. Metabolism, for instance, is more efficient when there is sufficient hydration to perform the Krebs Cycle (the sequence of reactions by which most cells release stored energy). Your body sends you an alert when your hydration levels are low by making you feel thirsty. Thirst is an alert for dehydration. If you ignore it, you run the risk of problems that can get much worse.

This can also happen when you run out of a specific minerals or nutrients – let's say iron, as a familiar example. When you run out of this nutrient, your body tries to give you a heads-up on what it needs, and you feel a sensation or an appetite or impulse to eat things like steak or other foods high in iron. In my own case, it manifests as the desire to have a steak; my wife will suddenly have a desire to eat scallops or clams. We all have different libraries of accumulated knowledge in our body to tell us which foods have been experienced as the best sources for specific nutrients. That "library" is something we build up over the course of our lives, and is based on the foods that we have gone out in the world and tried.

Unfortunately, recent generations face a major problem in making food choices. Their senses and appetites have been trained to point them in the wrong directions. If we have become generationally incapable of choosing the right foods, then how can we be expected to make the right choices?

The battle is really between opposing impulses from your brain/body. Your brain/body knows how to trigger your sense of thirst when you need more water. In the same way, it knows how to trigger your appetite for iron-rich foods when that need arises. At the same time, however, there is another part of your brain that is craving for a "fix," the kind of fix it gets whenever you eat junk food.

So, just what is "junk food"?

Junk food is anything that is engineered for taste but is deficient in nutrition.

Sugar cravings

Take, for instance, a tablespoon of normal table sugar. It is an amazing ingredient, convenient, cheap, and pleasing. The sweetness gives you a boost of glucose. But it has zero nutrients. All the nutrients the sugar had when it was first harvested from the cane or the beet have been stripped and bleached away to produce plain sugar. Processed white sugar gets addicting very fast. Just a little and the body's surge of energy is recorded in your biological library. A few more hits of sugar and the corresponding boost in energy is an established relationship. So, the next time you need energy, you are going to crave sugar. Have you ever been in a situation where you were stressed and you started to crave candy? When the body is under stress, it craves energy to prepare for fight or flight, and if those energy stores are depleted, you need to have something sweet to replenish it fast.

Salt cravings

Salt is something else your body naturally craves. Salt is a critical ingredient in the human body, maintaining the required salinity to aid in healthy diffusion and to keep the body's electrical conductivity at its peak.

If you want to understand the role of salt in the body's electrical conductivity, try this experiment when you get a chance. Take a pail of pure water. Put a battery beside the pail, and connect a wire from the negative lead to the positive terminal of lightbulb on the other side of the pail. Connect a second wire to the positive lead of the battery, dropping the other end into the water. Connect a third wire to the negative terminal of the lightbulb and drop the other end into the water. Now you have a positive lead from the battery in the water and a negative lead from the bulb in the water, but they aren't touching. What happens? Nothing.

Now, start adding a little salt and dissolve it in the water. You won't see any difference at first because there is too little salt, but as you keep adding more, you will gradually start to see the bulb light up. This happens because salt is an electrolyte, which increases the conductivity of water, and which, in turn, allows electrons to pass, completing the electrical circuit.

There are many electrical systems in your body – your heart is one of them. The impulses that run along your nerves from your brain to the rest of your body are also electrical in nature. All of these electrical systems need salt to function. For this and other reasons, salt is constantly craved by your body, and you are rewarded when you consume it. Many junk foods take advantage of the body's natural desire for salt.

Fat cravings

The third element the body craves almost as much as sugar is fat. Think of bacon, greasy fries, or moist roasts. Fat is something that the body rewards you for when you consume it. Later on, we'll be talking about why your body rewards you for eating fat.

So, let's take a closer look at the reasons for the body's desire to consume fat, bacon, chocolates, butter, and so on. Think back to our Paleolithic ancestors and consider what their basic patterns of consumption were and how their metabolism worked. They survived on a higher ratio of fat to carbohydrates than we do today. The largest part of their meal consisted of the meat that they hunted, and they gorged on that meat. Once that was done, and they had none left, they rested and hung around their dwellings. For the next 24 to 48 hours, they didn't hunt. If they felt the need, they would pick on berries and fruits. The ratio of protein and fat to carbs that they lived on was heavily in favor of the fat and proteins, which gave them tremendous energy and mental acuity. Our ancestors had so much energy that they could chase prey, and while they couldn't always catch them, they could keep on the chase until the prey was so exhausted it would give up or die from exhaustion.

It also gave them highly tuned instincts of what to eat, and they only ate when they were hungry or when there was an opportunity.

Fat was the energy store of choice, and it was also the preferred item on the menu. The metabolic chemistry of those early humans was very different than what we have today. While the underlying systems remain the same, we are forcing it to adapt to a different environment.

Our ancestors would eventually consume this fat, and when that fat was processed in the gut and transported to all areas around the body, hours after the meal, these hunter-gatherers slept and relaxed because their body was busy stocking up on the fuel source. About 1,000-1,400 calories would be stored as glycogen in the liver and skeletal muscles, while the rest was converted to fat in a process called lipogenesis.

During lipogenesis, excess calories are converted into triglycerides and carried via the bloodstream to be deposited in different areas. At that time, this was the primary source of energy. Carbohydrates was a backup source of energy and was used for the body's functions during the time the body was processing the food. It was also used to sustain the body while the food was converted to fat.

These hunter-gatherers lived a feast-or-famine lifestyle, so the body, which relied more on fat, had to also develop a parallel system of energy creation which was dependent on fast energy from carbs and proteins. Carbs and shorter chain sugars from fruits provided an instant pick-me-up for those who were feeling lethargic, but it would be a short-lived burst of energy. The sugars would be quickly mopped up and stored as fat or flushed out of the system. Nonetheless, it was a quick access to energy.

Once the lipogenesis process was complete, people could then go about their day and do what they had to. Once they had burned through their calories and were accessing their fat stores, they would be back to feeling hungry and went off on a hunt once again.

Habit-forming dopamine "hits"

Our ancestor's energy needs were primarily driven by fats, and so, even today, when we taste fat, we are rewarded with bliss.

We like these flavors because dopamine is released whenever we have foods that are engineered just right. Unfortunately, that dopamine release can go on to do something more insidious. Because dopamine release gives pleasure, that helps to create a habit. If you do something a few times and are rewarded for it each time, it becomes a habit. Eventually, you no longer have to think about it because it has become an automatic and habitual response.

The magic triumvirate

The triumvirate of ingredients, fat, salt, and sugar, are the magic ingredients of any manufactured or processed food. Major food manufacturers spend millions to research the best mix with just the right ratio of fat, sugar and salt to get the most people "hooked" on their products. Be it potato chips, sauces, candy bars, power drinks, soda, burgers, fast foods, or any other fast or processed food, the key is to get the consumer to come back for more. They do it by playing around with the flavor, especially combinations of fat, sugar, and salt, which are naturally powerfully attractive to humans and very addictive.

The first time you consume this deliciously-engineered food, the body gets its salt, sugar, and fat, and you are rewarded with a hit of dopamine. You like the reward of feeling great after eating the food, and so you try to repeat it, and you are rewarded again. A few more times, and you are hooked. Of course, everyone has the right to choose what they put into themselves – but just because mercury is freely available doesn't mean you should ingest it.

The silencing of true cravings

Not only do these "junk" food addictions steer you toward specific food items, but they also do something else much more insidious – they silence the true appetite cravings one might otherwise have. When you can't tell what your body is craving, you can't give it what it needs.

The more you eat the foods you are addicted to, the less the chance that you are getting the nutrients you really need, and so you feel hungry more often, and end up consuming more calories, and you can end up piling on the weight.

How does this really work? Well, when it's 'time' to have a meal, the first problem is that your body alerts you by giving you a sensation that it is hungry. That's typically not the right place to start from, because your body should only get hungry when it has no energy left in reserves. And unfortunately, when your senses are clouded, you are likely to crave the usual triumvirate of salt, sugar, and fat – in some form. And that is the problem.

Even when you may not need the calories (energy), hunger can be triggered by the body's nutritional needs. If, for example, your body needs potassium, and it is urgent, then, no matter how much you feed yourself, as long as that potassium (or some other mineral) is lacking, the body will keep sending you signals of being hungry. So, you run to the pantry to make a midnight snack, or head out to an all-night diner to satisfy that hunger. Whatever you do, you have just taken on extra calories, but are probably not any closer to getting the nutrients you actually need.

This is the core reason for the prevalence of obesity in America today. Even though that obesity is easily explained away as the result of the high fat content of fast food, and so on, the real reason isn't only that we overeat, it's also that we don't get the nutrients the body really needs so our hunger is never really satisfied.

The rest of this book is devoted to looking at how you can get rid of those addictive cravings. This is an advanced version of the intermittent fast, and, more importantly, it's a strategy to get healthier, not just slimmer. Eventually, it is possible to reach the stage where the body will only give you the appetite for what needs replenishing, whether that's energy or nutrients.

Chapter 2: Overview of the Intermittent Fast

Intermittent fasting returns you to the eating patterns of the generations that influenced your genetic makeup. That genetic inheritance established the forms of human metabolic functioning and set the order of energy creation.

Metabolism of Sugars and Fats

First, there is the metabolism of sugars through the process of glycolysis to create ATP, the molecule that stores and transports energy within cells. In glycolysis, one molecule of glucose is converted into carbon dioxide and two ATP molecules in the cytoplasm of a cell. The ATP is then used as energy in the cell for whatever it needs to do. Each molecule of glucose results in 2 ATP.

Second, there is the metabolism of fats, that is, the conversion of triglycerides, a type of fat (lipid) found in the blood and stored in fat cells. The conversion of one triglyceride molecule produces 406 ATP – more than 200 times the amount of ATP generated in glycolysis. This is one advantage of burning fat for energy instead of glucose.

When you are in a perpetual intermittent fast, your body is going to gradually switch to using triglycerides instead of glucose for energy more often.

Long distance runners are experts at achieving this switch from burning glucose to burning fats. They load up on food for days before a long-distance event, and then eat right before the event, filling up their reserves of glycogen. That glycogen in the liver and skeletal muscles amounts to about 1,000-1,400 calories. Long distance runners will burn through this fast once the marathon starts. A little later, when they have exhausted all their glycogen reserves, they will begin to burn fat. People who aren't used to this will feel an immense lethargy at the point the glycogen runs out. Some will even pass out. Seasoned pros, however, know how to get past "the wall."

Once the body starts converting triglycerides, there is a short lag, but the release of energy soon speeds up as it is more efficient than converting glucose. Once the metabolism has completely switched from the metabolism of glycogen to the metabolism of triglycerides, energy becomes abundantly available. The brain is then fed with ketones, instead of glucose, while the body starts to burn fat rapidly and effectively. The runner is then back up to speed, and can run extreme distances without stopping. The only thing they need is to constantly replenish their hydration. Without the necessary hydration, those metabolic processes will stall.

Easing into Intermittent Fasting

Just as you wouldn't expect to successfully start running extreme distances overnight, you can't really jump into intermittent fasting and hope to enjoy the benefits or the process right way. It is too much of a shock to the system, and there would be a system-wide revolt. This revolt manifests itself as headaches, mood swings, and lethargy. The better way is to ease into intermittent fasting. That is the reason for having a transitional induction week.

During induction week, the objective is to get your body ready for the process of shifting from relying on glucose and glycogen stores for all your energy needs into burning fat for energy. Do not take this lightly. Restoring your body's natural metabolic processes is supposed to be great, but if you do it too abruptly, at worst, it will mess with you unpredictably, or, at best, it is going to be so uncomfortable that you will give up and quit.

Once you have spent a week (or two weeks, if you need it) making the transition of induction week, you can move onto the initial fasting period. Not only will this free up a lot of your time normally spent eating and processing food, it will set you up for eating on a schedule that suits you or gets you into the rhythm of eating only when you genuinely need to.

Finally, you will get to the maintenance part of the diet. That is when you get your body off a rigid feeding schedules to arrive at your own schedule where you can confidently listen to your own body about when to eat. That will also be when you will figure out how much to eat, and what your appetites mean, so that you will know what you are really craving.

The next chapter is all about getting prepared for intermittent fasting during your induction week. We will look at the objectives that you have to set for yourself in both physical and psychological terms as well as the logistics of it. We will also look at establishing some good new habits and abandoning some bad ones, so that you can magnify the results of your intermittent fasting.

If you are ready, it is time to get started.

Chapter 3: Induction Week

Decide when you want to begin induction week – it should take you seven straight days. In my experience, going away for the weekend is a great time to get started, because it gets you away from things you tend to do by habit. If you try to start intermittent fasting surrounded by memory stimuli, such as your dining room and kitchen, then you will be constantly reminded to grab lunch or dinner at specific times, or to go back for snacks and junk food (assuming you are a snack lover).

The point of this first week is to expand your range of gastronomical choices and to cleanse the bodily systems that can make it harder to be on an intermittent fast.

The first thing you need to do this week is to remove all the processed foods from your diet, especially the fast foods, soda, and anything that comes pre-packaged or pre-seasoned. Your best bet is to eat fresh, organic food, but if you can't get organic food, don't worry, just make sure it's fresh. Otherwise, you can eat anything you want – steaks, dairy, fish, meat. It's all fair game here.

Day 0

On Day 0, you can really eat almost anything you want, whenever you want, with a few restrictions that will start cleansing your system. On Day 0, you want to cut out caffeine, soda, processed foods, junk food, fast foods, processed salt (you can substitute sea salt or Himalayan salt), and all sugar, and candy.

Also, drink fresh water throughout the day. Mineral water is fine but avoid reverse osmosis water which losses beneficial minerals and tends to be more acidic. Add two slices of lemon to a liter of water and drink that. When you have finished the first liter, use another two slices of lemon to a fresh bottle. In total, you are going to drink 2 liters of water.

Your last meal before starting the induction week of intermittent fasting will be on the evening of Day 0.

Stop eating at 7 p.m. on Day 0, but keep your water near you. If you finish your daily quota of 2 L of water, but you still feel like drinking more, go ahead. At night, however, the water you keep next to you should just be plain and clear water. You don't need to add the two slices of lemon to your nighttime water.

Day 1

On Day 1, you are going to perform a dawn-to-dusk fast where you don't eat anything and only consume water. Fill your water bottle again with water and lemon.

Go for a walk in the morning, and see the sights of wherever you are visiting for these first days of induction week. When you feel hungry, take a sip of water, but go out and take part in any activity that does not involve eating. Go have a blast – and forget about food.

One of the goals of Day 1 is to begin resetting your mental frameworks for the way you think about food, and for when you think of food. Everything about fasting and the habits of eating are more about mental issues than they are about physical or physiological ones. Your body is not going to crave food as much as your mind is.

Continue drinking water throughout the day until 7 p.m. when you will be having supper, your one meal of the day.

Ideally, you should arrive wherever you are going to have dinner a half hour early. Since you will be breaking fast at 7 p.m., get there at 6:30 and spend some time with your thoughts. Think over the day and how often you felt hunger and what exactly that was about. Feel free to make all the notes you need. Take these moments for evaluation because you need to become more sensitive to what your cravings and appetite signals are really telling you.

For dinner, start with some juice to stimulate your appetite and digestion. You can really have just about anything you want – just stay away from the processed and junk foods. At the end of your meal, you can even treat yourself to coffee and even ice cream – so long as it is not processed. Eat as much as you want, but make sure you are listening to your stomach (you know what I mean) instead of listening to your taste buds.

Feel the food, chew it, and savor the flavors. Separate the taste of the main ingredients from the spices. Get to know your food and take your time. Have the salad, have the meat or fish, whatever you want, and, with each item, make a mental note of how much you enjoy the food.

When you are done, realize that everything is really going well. You should be proud of yourself at this point. You have overcome your usual cravings and your body, no matter how weak you felt just before you broke fast, you were doing fine.

For the rest of the day, there are no more snacks to have or beverages to drink except water. When you go to bed, keep the bottle of water by your bedside.

Day 2

When you wake up on Day 2, start with your lemon water. Whether you decide to stay in, go out on the town, or get ready to head back for the work week ahead, remember you won't be eating anything during the day.

One of the things you will want to do is to prepare for breaking your fast at home. If you can, try to make dinner at home, or at least eat at home. If you don't have the supplies, the natural or unprocessed ingredients, you'll need to stock your pantry before you cook Day 2's meal. You don't really need to fill up your house with organic ingredients (If you can, that's great, but that can be expensive).

Remember, what's most important in intermittent fasting is the schedule of eating that you keep to. But you do want to drain your system of the chemicals typically found in processed foods, because that will help you enormously with intermittent fasting.

Cleansing the System of "Junk" Foods

There are sections of recipes and lists of foods scattered throughout this book to help you get started. The objective is to expand your "library" of nutritional sources, and to remove the hold that unhealthy ingredients in processed foods have on your habits and gastronomical pleasure centers. Most people do not fully appreciate just how many of their food choices are made "under the influence" of the choices that processed foods have predisposed them to. It's like giving a kid candy – after a while, that's all they want to eat because that candy has predisposed them to a sugary diet. In a similar way, processed foods predispose you to an unhealthy and inadequate diet.

Induction week is all about returning freedom of choice to you. Once you get rid of the toxins from your diet, they become less of a distraction as you move forward with intermittent fasting. Without the transition of the induction phase of the program, when you try to expand your food choices, the intermittent fast will become very difficult because of the addictions to salt, sugar, and fat and all the other ingredients in typical processed items, such as nitrates, hydrogenated oils, high fructose corn syrup, and flavor enhancers.

The focus of induction week is on cleansing the body of those habits and on flushing your system out as your body is rebalanced in the absence of the accumulated toxins. This will do two things for you. First, it stops the cravings for food when you are not really hungry. Second, it changes the kinds of food you crave, allowing you to have an appetite only for what your body actually needs.

Just be aware, the effort to remove the addiction to processed foods will be a tough one. But that is exactly what you need to do to make sure that you regain control and the power of choice. It is not that simple to scrub your addiction to a particular item. There are many ways to overcome an addiction, whether to nicotine, alcohol, opioids, food items, or anything else, but they are not always the same way, because the chemistry of addiction varies by substance. The severity of each addiction also differs, and therefore its hold and what it takes to overcome will also differ.

The addiction to processed foods can be severe, at best. Food is a matter of life and death and the brain sees the lack of it as a threat to existence. And even more in the modern world is the idea of stopping food simply scorned. However, fasting for a day overcomes this fallacy, and serves to cleanse the chemical echoes that cause the difficulty.

Caloric needs and addictive cycles

All of your food intake will fall into one of two categories: first, what satisfies your caloric needs for the day, and, second, what satisfies the nutritional needs of the day.

Caloric needs are those needs you have for the energy all cells need to function. Without energy, nothing works. For this reason, the brain is designed to seek out energy and to calculate how much energy it needs. The brain sees taking in calories as the ultimate security feature. Without energy, the brain becomes dysfunctional and then the body dies. Because it is so important, any time energy is given to the body, you are rewarded with a rush of dopamine, and that, in turn, creates a habit. Children are especially susceptible to this habit-forming cycle, because they need loads of energy to fuel their activities and growth, yet they have a small gastrointestinal capacity.

PH balance, digestion and nutrients

Adding lemon to your drinking water starts to change the acidity of your internal chemistry. Not only does the lemon help maintain your body's electrolyte balance, but lemon is an incredible fruit with unconventional acid-alkaline properties. Usually, when you ingest something acidic, like vinegar, it enters your system and remains acidic. It has an acidic bias in your blood chemistry. That makes sense – if it is acidic outside, it's acidic inside. But this is not so with the lemon you add to your drinking water. Lemon has the uncanny ability to change from acid to alkaline once it is digested in the body. It's net effect on your digestive system and then your blood is to make it mildly alkaline.

The human body, itself, has a variety of pH profiles. Acid levels in the stomach, for instance, are between 2 and 3.5 pH. This is the reason you have a mucosal layer to protect the tissues of the stomach from erosion by the acids secreted during the digestive process. When the digested food (called chyme) leaves the stomach, it is highly acidic at about 2 pH, and that is not a good thing for the digestive tract. The digestive tract is a porous sheath that allows water to carry the released nutrients across its membrane to the network of blood vessels that encapsulates its entire length. To counter the inhospitable acidity, the duodenum releases *cholecystokinin*, a hormone that signals the gallbladder to reduce the acidity by releasing bile which is highly alkaline. By the time the chyme passes to the rest of the small intestine, it is at a neutral or even slightly alkaline pH. That permits efficient absorption of nutrients across the membrane and into the blood.

One side effect of eating processed foods is to raise acid levels in the body. The few days you stop eating the heavily processed foods that cause acid-forming substances to accumulate, while drinking lemon water to counteract the acidity of the digestive environment, will make a huge difference in the way your body functions, and how effectively nutrients are absorbed.

Nutrition density vs. calories

The more effectively you absorb the nutrients your body needs, the less calories (energy) you will need to ingest. Remember the duality of all the foods we consume – calories versus nutrients. Let's be clearer about that. Everything you ingest has calories. Even if you chewed paper up and swallowed it, it will have a caloric value. Whether you eat beef to get the iron you need, or eat salmon, aside from the taste, the difference lies in the number of calories you take in as you get your iron. This is referred to as nutrition density. On the one hand, substances like table sugar have zero nutrition but a high number of calories. On the other hand, foods like broccoli have lots of nutrients and low calories.

Processed foods that create addictive cycles are low ratio items, meaning that they have high amounts of calories but low levels of nutrients. So, while you get more than the amount of energy you need for the day, you aren't getting enough of the nutrients, micronutrients, and vitamins the body needs to replenish itself. Energy is just one part of the equation. All the energy in the world is not going to help you pedal a bicycle if your muscles are not functioning properly as the result improper tissue maintenance caused by a lack of the right nutrients.

The following is a list of examples of foods that have a high nutrient density. You should try to include as many of these kinds of foods as you can during the induction period.

- Beef Liver

- Salmon

- Broccoli

- Kale

- Shellfish

- Potatoes

- Sardines

- Garlic

- Seaweed

- Dark Chocolate

You want to start resetting your body's "library" of food choices to include foods with a high nutrition density so that you take in the greatest amount of nutrients for the least number of calories. Given the opportunity, your body can start recognizing and craving nutrient rich foods. You are certainly not required to eat these foods exclusively, but eating more nutrient dense food, in itself, will begin to help you drop any unwanted weight.

How unsatisfied nutritional hunger piles on calories

Let's look at the way that unsatisfied cravings for nutrients can cause you to eat more calories than you need.

Let's say your body is telling you that it is hungry and that you have an appetite for beef liver, something in your body's nutrient "library." There is a good chance that something like iron or B-complex is in deficit in your body – which is normal – it just needs to be replenished. But instead of frying up some liver, you decide to reach for that extra-large slice of cheesecake. Initially, it fills you up, you feel good, and you have taken on 400 calories. Once your stomach has gone through processing that cheesecake, your system recognizes that the nutrients it needs are still not there, so it sends another signal to your brain that it needs liver, but you still don't give it liver. Instead, you fill up on a peanut butter sandwich. There's another 150 calories. Now you are up to 550 calories, and your body still hasn't received what it has been asking for.

By this point, you're very hungry, so you head over to your favorite diner, and finally have that plate of liver and onions. It hits the spot, but you now have added another 400 calories. You are no longer hungry, but you've taken on a total of 950 calories. If you had just listened to your body, and got what it was asking for all along, you wouldn't have eaten that extra 550 calories. Extrapolate this pattern out over a week, or an entire year, and you can easily see why two out of three North American adults are either overweight or obese.

There are all sorts of diets that don't account for the body's nutritional requirements and focus only on calories. This is counterproductive, both for losing the excess weight, and for being healthy.

Intermittent fasting is about changing the frequency of your meals to suit your metabolic profile. However, by also paying attention to your nutritional needs, you can learn to let your body to tell you when it is hungry only when it has real nutritional needs, instead of piling on calories that are beyond what it needs for energy.

Processed foods vs. your body's "library" of nutritional sources

Processed foods also diminish the efficacy of the intermittent fast in another way. Suppose you ate a fast food burger, taking in all the salt, sugar and fat that went with it, and you feel good. The problem is that it is nutritionally deficient, right? Yes, but it is worse than that.

That burger does have some nutrition, so the body records this food item in its "library" as a possible source for the nutrients it needs. So, let's say a fast food burger supplies 20% of your daily B12 requirement but also supplies 400 calories – you would need five burgers to reach that daily B12 requirement. That's 2,000 calories that you would have to take in. Compare that to a fresh serving of lightly grilled salmon that is only about 250 calories yet supplies 100% of your daily B12 requirement.

If you only expose yourself to fast food burgers, your body will believe that the burger is the only source of B12, so every time you need B12, your cravings will direct you to that fast food burger. However, when you introduce a great tasting freshly grilled and nutrient-packed salmon, especially during induction week when you have stopped all processed food, your body will begin to update the records in its nutritional "library," especially after a number of repetitions of the experience. Eventually when you need B12, you'll experience a hankering for grilled salmon, instead of the burger with its unnecessary extra calories.

Summary of Goals for Induction Week

During this intermittent fasting program, the objectives of induction week are to:

- Ease the addictive hold of processed foods,

- Increase the variety of fresh foods in your diet,

- Improve the nutritional density of your food,

- Improve the alkaline/acid balance of your body, and

- Drink plenty of water.

Day 3

On Day 3, you are probably back at work after your weekend, and you should start your day with a brisk walk. An average of a 30-minute walk around the block is a great way to start your day. The increased metabolism from walking and the increased oxygen intake from the fresh morning air will go a long way toward getting your metabolism working.

Turning fat-burning metabolism "on"

At this point, it won't be your regular metabolism – the one that burns glucose and glycogen – that is kicking into gear, it will be the metabolism that uses triglycerides. That means you will be burning fat. Once you start burning fat, every minute of workout you do has an impact on your weight loss objective or at least contributes to your overall effort.

The average person burns about 1,800 to 2,200 calories per day (women) and 2,800 to 3,200 calories per day (men). Those ranges take into account overall lifestyle. The higher calorie burn numbers are for those with active lifestyles, and the lower numbers are for those who are less active.

When you sleep, you burn about 0.42 calories per pound of body weight per hour of sleep. So, let's say you are 180 pounds and sleep 8 hours a night. You can calculate that by multiplying 0.42 by your weight in pounds by the number of hours you sleep. In this example, that would work out as 0.42 x 180 x 8 or 605 calories. That's just when you sleep.

When you wake up and go out for your 30-minute walk in the morning, you are going to burn approximately 200 calories. By the time you hit the showers in the morning, you have already used up 800 calories. Remember that your body only stores about 1,400 calories in the liver and the skeletal muscles. Once that has been used up, the body will have to switch metabolic engines and begin to burn fat stores instead.

When you get to work, even if you are sitting all day, you are burning about 70 calories per hour. Over the entire day, that's 700 calories (on the low side). So, now, you are already up to about 1,500 calories, past the body's glycogen stores (unless you consume food along the way). That means you will come to a point where you feel tired, and then, a little while later, you will feel an energy surge as the triglycerides start being converted for energy. Once you start burning fat for energy, you will notice how powerful and alert you feel.

Although the body does well burning fat as fuel, it can't do it all on fat-based energy. You are not limiting your food sources, except for avoiding refined sugar and processed food. When you eat anything you feel like, you will find that you end up getting any carbohydrates you need as well as the nutrients. The carbohydrates you take in will provide the glucose the brain needs, which is about 20% of total fuel. If you can feed your brain that ratio of 80:20, you will start to see an uptick in mental performance.

During induction week, you are getting your body to experiment with repeated switching between fuel sources. Your body has been accustomed to using glucose and glycogen as its primary energy source. In the beginning, fasting will feel hard, because your body has forgotten how to switch from glycogen to triglycerides. But it will remember when it is pushed. You just have to hold fast.

During induction week, you will have triggered triglyceride metabolism at least once every day, and that will create a visceral memory of how to do it at a moment's notice. It will also fine-tune the process so that it triggers and stabilizes faster. By the time you get to intermediate week, your body should have become more proficient at making the change quickly. It won't be perfect, but it will be getting there.

Days 3 to 7

For days 3 to 7, the schedule will stay the same through the rest of the week.

Every day, go for that brisk walk in the morning, for about 30 minutes. If you have a treadmill, that's great, but try to get out to breathe the fresh morning air. It really does make a difference.

You won't eat anything throughout the day, so at lunchtime, if you are in an office or other work environment, try to politely excuse yourself from the lunch crowd, and go to the park or a museum instead. If you have the energy, go to the gym. But whatever you do, stay away from friends who are eating. The idea is to keep your mind off of food and the usual schedule for eating. You have a deeply entrenched habit of eating at lunchtime. You need to jettison that habit and being around people who are eating lunch is not going to help.

Later, when you get home, you can eat almost anything you want to, but stick to these simple guidelines:

1.   No processed food or ingredients,

2.   No sugar, and

3.   No fast foods.

Keep drinkable water with a slice of lemon with you at all times. Take a sip anytime you feel a little dry in the mouth, or you think you feel hungry.

One of the things you will notice is that your urine will become clear after the second or third day. Proper hydration, plus a little bit more, will be helping to flush accumulated toxins, and the electrolytes from the lemon will balance the salinity of the systems in your body.

At the end of this transitional induction week, evaluate whether you need to go a day or more than the seven days that you have already done. How would you know? That will vary from one person to the next. If you have found it getting easier for you to stick to one meal a day, it means your body has started to get the proper nutrients, and that your metabolism has become more adaptable. If you feel this is true, then it will be time to move on to the next phase, intermediate week.

12 Recipes

The following are some recipes to inspire you to the kind of eating you want to take you through induction week. You aren't required to eat these foods. These recipes are only provided here to make it easier for you. This is not like some other diets where the routine is fixed.

Whatever you eat, keep the ingredients fresh and unprocessed. This will help flush your system of toxins and chemicals while adding to your body's personal "library" of foods that do your body good. Once your body starts to feel really good, it will begin to prefer this type of food over others, and your body will like the feeling of staying light and active with the new eating schedule.

Grilled Salmon

2 lbs. (900 g) side of salmon (skin on)

½ teaspoon fine sea/Himalayan salt

½ teaspoon ground black pepper

8 teaspoons extra virgin olive oil

3 teaspoons mixed fresh herbs (tarragon, marjoram, thyme, and parsley), chopped

olive oil

juice of 3 lemons

Clean salmon with cool running water. Pat dry. Rub the sea salt into the fish and wrap with three layers of clean disposable kitchen towels. This will extract the moisture from the salmon. Set aside for 10 minutes.

Using a mortar and pestle, grind the herbs, pepper, and olive oil into a runny paste.

Remove the disposable towels from the salmon, leaving the salt that has stuck to the fish. Using your hands, rub the oil/pepper/herb paste all over the salmon.

Use additional olive oil to grease a heated grill. Cook the salmon on the grill for about 15 minutes. You only need to flip it once or three times.

Drizzle salmon with lemon juice before serving.

Yield: 8 servings

Beetroot Feta Salad

2 oz. (60 g) cooked beetroot, cubed

1 oz. (30 g) feta cheese, cubed

2 oz. (60 g) spinach, blanched

lemon

sea salt

ground black pepper

Toss beetroot, feta cheese, and spinach together. Squeeze the lemon over it. Add sea salt and pepper to taste.

Yield: 1 serving

Mexican Sausage Delight

1 Mexican chorizo sausage (2.8 oz.) (80 g)

2 Italian sausages (2.8 oz.) (80 g)

2 large eggs

1 small red onion, diced

1 jalapeno pepper, chopped

1 teaspoon paprika

3 tablespoons extra virgin olive oil

juice from 1 fresh lime

juice from 1 fresh lemon

juice from 3 fresh calamondin lime

sea salt

ground black pepper

1 teaspoon fresh oregano

1 cup cherry tomatoes, quartered

1 red bell pepper, chopped

1 medium spring onion, chopped

1 large avocado, diced

2 teaspoons fresh coriander

sour cream

Poach eggs in boiling salted water. Use a slotted spoon to remove the eggs from the water. Set the eggs aside on a kitchen towel to absorb excess water. Season the eggs with sea salt and pepper to taste.

De-case the sausages and fry the meat in a dry pan until the meat browns and cooks. It should take no longer than 6 minutes. Add the red onions and jalapenos and continue to cook, stirring until the onions soften. Sprinkle with paprika. Reduce heat to medium and continue frying until the meat turns a darker shade of brown. Remove from heat.

Combine olive oil, juices from the lemons and limes, salt, and pepper in a separate bowl. Add tomatoes, oregano, peppers, avocado, and spring onion. Toss it all together to make a simple salsa.

To serve, start with the meat and place the egg on top of it. Top all with the salsa mix, then add the sour cream and coriander.

Yield: 2 servings

Sweet Plums & Yogurt

3.5 oz. (100 g) natural yogurt

2 plums, pitted and chopped

1 tsp. of honey

Combine and serve.

Yield: 1 serving

Turkey Patties

turkey, minced

small egg, beaten

spring onion, chopped

garlic

chili powder to taste

Mix the egg in with the turkey, spring onion, garlic, and chili. Discard extra egg, if any.

Form the mixture into patties. Fry patties on a grill.

Yield: 1 serving

Roast Vegetables with Balsamic Vinegar

1 roasted zucchini (courgette)

1 roasted eggplant (aubergine)

1 roasted butternut squash

1 roasted red pepper

1 tbsp. balsamic vinegar

juice of 1 lemon

Chop and slice all.

Combine all together with the lemon juice and balsamic vinegar.

Yield: 1-2 servings

Hummus with Vegetables

1 cup hummus

carrots, chopped

cucumber, chopped

green and/or red pepper, chopped

edamame beans

rock salt

Steam vegetables and edamame. Add salt. Spoon over hummus.

Yield: 1-2 servings

Turkey Breasts & Spinach

1 turkey breast steak

1 tablespoon clarified butter

1 cup cooked spinach

sea salt

Melt butter in skillet. Fry turkey breast.

Serve turkey over bed of spinach seasoned with salt.

Yield: 1 serving

Pita Pizza Wrap

whole meal pita

Philadelphia cream cheese

1 tomato, chopped

mixed herbs

sea salt

ground black pepper

Spread cream cheese over pita. Sprinkle with tomato, herbs, salt, and pepper. Fold to serve.

Yield: 1 serving

Aioli

6 cloves fresh garlic, peeled

2 tablespoons extra virgin olive oil

dash sea salt

¼ lemon

To make aioli, blend all ingredients above in a food processor to a smooth paste. If you have a large food processor, you'll need to make more; just multiply the quantities given, keeping the ratio of ingredients as above.

Use in recipes as directed.

Aioli Chicken with Vegetable Couscous

1 chicken breast

1 tablespoon aioli paste (see above)

3.5 oz. (100 g) vegetable couscous, cooked

Coat chicken with aioli. Grill the chicken. Mound couscous on the grilled chicken, and serve.

Yield: 1 serving

Roasted Red Pepper & Chicken Soup

7 oz. (200 g) chicken, cubed

1 chicken stock cube

4 cups water

½ roasted red pepper, chopped

½ roasted tomato, chopped

½ roasted onion, chopped

1 clove garlic, chopped

1 tsp. tomato puree

½ tsp. cumin

½ tsp. balsamic vinegar

sea salt

ground black pepper

Boil the chicken and stock cube in a pot of water. Remove the chicken and set aside.

Add the rest of the ingredients to the pot. Use a stick blender to puree until smooth. Return the chicken pieces to the pot and serve.

Yield: 2 servings

Shopping List

In addition to ingredients from the recipes, you can use this as a shopping list and keep ingredients from it on standby in your pantry.

Oils

avocado oil
clarified butter (ghee)
coconut oil

cod liver oil
flax oil
olive oil

Beans, etc.

lentils
quinoa

Nuts and Seeds

almonds
cashews
chestnuts
pumpkin seeds
sesame seeds
sunflower seeds

Herbs, Spices, and Condiments

apple cider vinegar
basil
bay leaves
black pepper
cayenne pepper
cilantro
cinnamon
garlic
ginger root
parsley
sea salt
soy sauce
umeboshi vinegar (plum vinegar)

Fruits

apples
apricots
avocados
bananas
blackberries
blueberries
cantaloupe
cherries
coconut
grapefruit
grapes
honeydew melon
lemons
limes
nectarines
olives, green
oranges
papaya
pears
peaches
persimmon
pineapple
raisins
raspberries
strawberries
tangerines
watermelon

Vegetables

artichokes
asparagus
beets
bell peppers
broccoli
brussels sprouts
cabbage
carrots
cauliflower
celery
collard greens
cucumbers
eggplant
endive
kale
kohlrabi
mushrooms
mustard greens
okra
onions
parsnips
potatoes
snow peas
string beans
summer squash
sweet potatoes
yams
winter squash
zucchini

Extras

apple juice
ginger tea
grape juice
grapefruit juice
green/herbal tea
mineral water
molasses
orange juice
pineapple juice
raw cane sugar
rice syrup
wild rice

Chapter 4: Intermediate Week

Congratulations! You have just graduated to the intermediate week of this intermittent fasting program. Those periods of fasting should have been getting easier. You really need to pat yourself on the back. This past week is a real accomplishment. You have not only put your body through a tough week, you have also trained your mind to stay strong in the face of a great challenge.

Objectives for Intermediate Week

Now, your objective will be to focus your efforts on triggering fat metabolism. That is your yardstick.

During the coming week, the objective will be to lengthen the gaps between food on some days, and to have longer pockets of time to eat rather than to fill up in one meal. This will allow you to eat smaller quantities, while your body spends less time eating and more time doing other things, such as strengthening your immune system.

The objective of this week is to shorten the cycles of switching between the energy sources. You want the body to learn to adapt to a faster process of switching to burning fat for energy. For those of you looking to lose weight, or have aesthetic motives in mind, this is good news. If you are looking to do this for mental clarity, or simply to get healthier, burning fat is also good news for you. During your intermediate week of intermittent fasting, you should start to experience some positive effects. You will feel brighter, clearer, and more alert; you will start to feel more energy; and you will start to find that you are losing weight.

The point of intermittent fasting is to get the body functioning at optimal levels and to the full potential it has evolved to. Using energy from triglycerides (fats) is like using nitrous oxide in a car. It boosts both your body and your mind. If you happen to have fat to spare from years of accumulation, you will also lose the weight and feel better for it.

But what are you going to burn once you have used up (or don't have) excess weight? That is where you start taking on a high-fat content diet. This may sound counter-intuitive to generations who have been told that fat is unhealthy. Certainly, unnatural fat is bad for you, but natural animal-based fat is good for you. If you are vegan or vegetarian, there are alternatives to animal-based fats that you can consume if you are looking to burn fat for fuel. There is a section for vegans and vegetarians later in this chapter.

Cholesterol and Intermittent Fasting

We can't really talk about deliberately eating fats without talking about cholesterol. In fact, understanding cholesterol is a key to understanding how fat metabolism works in the body and in intermittent fasting.

Practitioners of intermittent fasting are likely to see changes in their cholesterol profiles during intermediate week, so this is a good time to address the issue of cholesterol.

How is your cholesterol level? Have you had it checked recently? Are you concerned about cholesterol? Do you intentionally avoid foods that contain cholesterol? You may think that fat and cholesterol are unhealthy and will lead to coronary problems. But that isn't really an accurate picture. Before you keep going on that track, there are some things that you need to know.

First, you need to understand that your body needs cholesterol. It is a critical lipoprotein without which we would not survive. Cholesterol is needed by cells – it is what is used to make cell membranes. It is also what is used to make the protective sheath protecting your nerves.

Cholesterol also aids in the production of some of the most important hormones in your body, including progesterone and estrogen. You don't even need to ingest cholesterol-rich foods to have cholesterol in your blood – your liver already makes plenty.

Lipids

A lipid is a general classification that includes different kinds of cholesterol, monoglycerides, diglycerides, triglycerides, fatty acids, and more. Lipids are biomolecules that cannot be dissolved in water or water-based liquids, including blood. Putting lipids into blood would be like pouring oil into water.

Earlier, we talked about triglycerides, a lipid, being moved through the bloodstream. Since lipids, on their own, are not water-soluble, they need to be attached to a protein to make them soluble in water – these are called lipoproteins. In other words, the lipids found in your circulatory system are floating around in the form of lipoproteins. Specifically, lipoproteins are found in your blood in five different forms of cholesterol.

5 types of cholesterol

The five types of cholesterol include the HDL and LDL forms that most people have heard of, but there are three more, including chylomicrons, VLDL and IDL. VLDL is an acronym for Very Low-Density Lipoprotein, and IDL stands for Intermediate Density Lipoprotein.

Let's look at each of them briefly.

High Density Lipoproteins (HDLs) move triglycerides to the liver for excretion. HDLs are considered good cholesterols.

Chylomicrons are made in the gastrointestinal tract. They carry the triglycerides made from the food you eat and that are being transported around the body. After a meal, there are higher levels of chylomicrons in the blood.

Very Low-Density Lipoproteins (VLDLs) are like chylomicrons in that they also carry triglycerides. However, VLDLs are created in the liver rather than the gastrointestinal track. VLDLs are packets of lipids that circulate to tissues where they are extracted. Once the triglyceride has been extracted by the cell, what is left is called an IDL.

Intermediate Density Lipoproteins (IDLs) are what's left once the triglycerides have been extracted, in part or in full, by the adipose tissue in the cardiac, skeletal muscles, as well as the subcutaneous layer. While the chylomicrons and VLDL are at high levels after a meal, after a few hours, the IDLs are higher, once the triglycerides have been deposited at their destinations around the body.

Low-Density Lipoproteins (LDLs) were once IDLs, but, after even more lipids have been extracted from them, they are reduced to being more shell than lipid. Remember that lipoproteins are lipids wrapped in protein shells for the purpose of transporting them through an aqueous solution. In the case of LDLs, most or all of those lipids have already been deposited in tissues all over the body. LDLs are considered the "bad" cholesterols.

Metabolic Momentum and Weight Loss

You should lose more weight this week. But that will only happen if you satisfy two prerequisites. First, continue drinking the 2 liters of lemon water. Second, walk for at least 30 minutes, briskly, first thing in the morning. Do it first thing in the morning, not later, not in the evening - but in the morning. Even if you are already in the practice of going to the gym, you still need to do this walk in the morning. During induction and intermediate weeks, you can't replace the walking with going to the gym.

Momentum is one reason you start losing weight. We face momentum in everything we do. Most things that are not the subject of effort are the physical manifestations of momentum, and this applies to all aspects of life – physical or conceptual. It's just like a car that you can accelerate to 100 km/h by flooring the gas, and once at 100 km/h, you can coast at that speed using a lot less gas. Momentum is the force that carries you forward.

Weight loss occurs when you gain metabolic momentum. When you constantly rely on glucose to fuel your daily physical and mental activities, you create a metabolic momentum that is in constant search for and use of glucose. Then, when you are out of energy, when that tank is empty, you instinctively search for glucose-heavy foods. In time, that becomes a habit. Unfortunately, when the body is driven by the metabolic momentum of using glucose, it starts a series of chain events that can destroy the body.

If the body starts supplying energy using fats and proteins instead, the body becomes more efficient. There are no insulin spikes, and no possibility of insulin resistance. You can build up a metabolic momentum to burn fat for energy instead.

Of course, you will still eat some carbohydrates along the way, and that is a good thing. This is not like the Atkins diet with its strict effort to stick only to proteins and fats, and its concerns about interrupting ketosis (metabolism of burning fat). No. In this intermittent fasting approach, you do want to include some carbohydrates in your diet. You want fats and proteins too – you basically want all things in your meal – if your body calls for them. There is no exclusion of food groups. The only thing to stop completely are processed foods.

Freeing up energy for more

Part of the momentum your body is developing is to devote more energy to the other processes of living life. It is about balance; your body needs the energy to do a variety of things beyond eating.

84

If you spend your day eating every few hours, then, those of you who are a little more advanced in age will recognize that your body starts to slow down after a meal, perhaps even nodding off. If you are younger, you might also have this problem, but you have certainly observed it in older folks. Those in their forties and fifties typically slow down after a meal. If they don't have coffee or caffeine in any form after a meal, they may come to a grinding halt.

This occurs because it takes a lot of energy resources for the body to digest and transport nutrients across the full length and breadth of the body. Numerous processes are at work in digestion and in circulating and moving nutrients. While this is going on, other systems are intentionally slowed down. Blood is directed away from the brain and limbs toward the length of the gut to extract and absorb nutrients and to move everything around.

When we eat every few hours through the day, the body has hardly any time to do anything else. One of the most important and beneficial things the body could be doing instead of constantly dealing with digestive processes is energizing the immune system to maintain the body's defenses.

Over the last five years, I have conducted two 30-day fasts which were very different in experience and outcome. The first was not only the most fulfilling and invigorating, it was also an eye-opener. One of the things that happened was that several scars on my leg from bike accidents faded. I had expected it, having read of others experiencing that, but it was still a breathtaking experience. More research, hours of conversations with fasting practitioners, and sessions with doctors helped me to understand why those scars disappeared.

Imagine it this way: if you hire a housekeeper to cook and clean for you, there are tasks in the house that you can delegate to your helper while you go out and take care of business. If you don't eat at home on most days, this helper will have to do fewer chores related to cooking and cleaning up after meals. With the focus on keeping the home clean, you would see a lot of cleaning done. The house would be tidy and spotless. Even the smallest of issues and details, like dust on door hinges, are likely to be taken care of.

However, if you started to stay at home more, only leaving for meals, that same helper would now be spending some of their time cleaning up after you. It would add a little to their routine, but there would still be lots of time to do the regular cleaning. Some of the finer cleaning details may take a hit, but, for the most part, all would still be well.

Now let's take this a few steps further. Suppose that not only do you begin to eat at home, with your helper doing all the cooking and after-meal clean-up, but you also have started eating every few hours. By the time you have finished one meal and the helper has cleaned up after it, it's almost time to start preparing the next meal. Most of the helper's time is now spent in the kitchen or running to the store for food. How is the rest of the house going to get cleaned? At best, you are going to run the helper ragged. Some chores would certainly get shelved and not done at all, tasks would begin to pile up, dust in the crevices would build up, and the house would start to fall into disarray.

I think you can see where I am going with this. The same thing happens with the resources in your body. When your body has to manage the intake of nutrients and the processes of moving them around, other functions have to be put on hold. The body automatically directs the use of resources according to a built-in priority system. For example, digestive processes stop instantly when fight or flight alarms are activated in the body, because digestion is a less immediate survival priority. On the other hand, digestion is given priority over other functions when the body's resources are managed.

Energy to clean up LDL cholesterol

One of the other things that happened to me after my first 30-day fast was that my LDL (the bad cholesterol) levels plummeted. That and the clearing of my scars are related in a common way.

Recall that there are five major types of cholesterol, and that cholesterol is just another word for bags of fat on their way to storage sites around the body.

When you eat, glucose is released to power the body, glycogen is stored in the liver and muscles to power the body for about half a day, and the rest is converted to fat, ready for longer term storage. Those triglycerides (fats) are packaged and prepared for distribution to different areas of the body. Since triglycerides need to be packaged in a protein sheath to be soluble in blood, those protein bags act like the bags you get when you go to the grocery store. Now imagine that your bloodstream is teeming with these bags of triglycerides on their way to different destinations in the body. Once a bag arrives at a particular place, it unloads some of those triglycerides, then it moves on to another location and unloads some more.

Once the bags have been effectively emptied, they become low-density lipoproteins (LDLs), with very low amounts of lipids in the protein bag. These are like the empty plastic bags that get tossed away onto the street after use. They enter the drainage system, blocking it, causing street flooding, and other problems. In the same way, those proteins sheets remain in the blood and accumulate over time. They start to form plaque which causes hardening and congestion of the arteries.

However, if the body is not constantly digesting food and shunting energy and fats around, it can shift into clean-up and repair mode. It can repair scars and remove unrecognized or unwanted tissue, such as LDLs. That's what happened to me during my fast, as my body redirected its time and energy to restoring my system, as good as new.

Stimulating Hormones with Fasting

The body is a powerful mechanism with the ability to keep the body stable by altering various hormones and regulating mechanisms. When it comes to fasting, there are three hormones, in particular, that you should know about – cortisol, noradrenalin, and HGH (human growth hormone).

Cortisol is a hormone with multiple purposes and it is part of the cocktail of elements released by the adrenal glands when a person stops eating during intermediate fasting or extended fasting. Among other things, cortisol regulates and controls

- blood pressure,
- the use of carbs, fats, and proteins,
- inflammation,
- blood glucose, and
- the sleep cycle.

Noradrenalin is also released. It is primarily involved in maintaining the homeostasis of the body and keeping the body's balance under all circumstances. Together with cortisol, noradrenalin is involved with returning the body to normal levels. The release of noradrenalin helps with the body's ability to return itself to the way the body was designed to be. Periods of fasting kickstarts this process.

Finally, HGH, human growth hormone, is the most important for our discussion. Human growth hormone is made by the pituitary gland. Deficiencies in HGH can lead to higher body fat retention, and decreased lean body mass and reduced bone mass. Fasting triggers HGH, so fasting is one way to counter those effects.

HGH lasts mere minutes after its release before it is metabolized by the liver and broken down into other compounds and hormones. One of these is IGF1 (insulin-like growth factor 1).

In natural and regular cycles, IGF1 is released by the body 2-3 hours before your regular wake up time. This was a curious finding, but it was eventually explained as the body, which is in a habit of waking up at a certain time, preparing for a boost of energy. So, if you are usually up by 7 a.m., you will get a shot of IGF1 at around 4 a.m. This explains why breakfast isn't the necessity that myth would have it be, and why you are still able to go for the morning walk even when you are fasting.

The human growth hormone plays a huge role in the regeneration and replacement of your bones, muscles and other tissue. Stimulating HGH during consistent periods of fasting allows your body to enjoy the benefits of the hormone without becoming immune to it. HGH also has an impact on the brain, both in terms of regeneration and creation of new neurons.

Intermediate Week Plan

During intermediate week, you should plan for longer fasting gaps with 4-hour eating "windows." This means that you can eat smaller portions more frequently during those eating windows rather one large meal.

You should also start to consume more fat and protein and fewer carbohydrates in your diet.

Make sure to have between 7 to 9 hours of sleep every night. Wake up no later than 7 a.m. and get out for your morning walk. This gets your body performing at a level that is healthy, expresses necessary hormones, and allows your metabolism to peak at a level that is constantly burning energy.

Make your morning walk a brisk one. If you were doing about 4 miles per hour last week, this week up it to about 4.5 mph and increase it to 45 minutes.

During your eating "windows," you will have 4 hours to eat whatever you want, but in smaller quantities. Then stop eating until the next eating "window," consuming only water with your trusty wedge of lemon.

There are three different eating schedules during intermediate week. Each will have a significant impact on how you adapt to this new approach to energy management. During induction week, you have already fasted for seven days having just one meal a day, so adapting to this more rigorous regime should be significantly easier.

Remember that the eating "windows" are open for 4 hours, so you can arrange your eating as you see fit.

The first of the three plans, Day 1 (D1), is to have one meal in the evening after 7 p.m. Do not have any food prior to this all day. Only have the water to drink. Arrange your day so that after you have consumed your meal, you can relax for the rest of the evening and then go off to sleep.

For that evening meal, you can choose from any of recipes in this chapter. You aren't limited to those, but I urge you to look through them to see the type of food suggested. Have a full meal, and you can have one, two, or three servings.

For Day 2 (D2), do not eat at all. Only water. Continue to go for your daily walks and have a normal day. Do what you would otherwise do, but make sure that you stay away from the kitchen. We eat more with our minds than with our stomach.

On Day 3 (D3), you will not eat anything in the morning, but you will have a good lunch. You can eat as many portions as you feel – but do not overeat. Do not think that you should load up just so you can fast longer. It doesn't work that way. Eat what you can and stop when you are full. Choose whatever you feel like having – only make sure that it's not processed food or items containing sugar. You will still need to consume at least 2L of water daily. There are no other meals on D3.

Again on Day 4 (D4), you will cleanse your system by not eating anything.

On Day 5 (D5), have a good breakfast after your walk. Don't think of it as breakfast – have a full meal, two portions if you like and if your body demands it. But don't persuade yourself that you should eat more than your body really needs. Don't eat until you are stuffed. Eat what you need, then stop.

Again, don't eat anything on Day 6 (D6).

Have another lunch or afternoon meal on Day 7 (D7).

Meal	1	2	3	4	DAY 5	6	7
Morning	0	0	0	0	MD5	0	0
Afternoon	0	0	AD3	0	0	0	AD7
Evening	ED1	0	0	0	0	0	0

ED1 – Evening Day 1

AD3 – Afternoon Day 3

MD5 – Morning Day 5

AD7 – Afternoon Day 7

Adding Fruit to Meals

You can add a boost by having a portion of fruits with each meal or during any eating "window." The following would be ideal, but any fruit with a pH between 3 and 4.5 works well.

Fruit	Glycemic Index	pH
Apples	39	3.6
Cherries	20	4.3
Dried Apricot	32	3.3
Grapefruit	25	3.5
Grapes	53	3
Peaches	42	3.5
Pears	38	4
Strawberries	41	3.5

Although fruits (and vegetables) may have an acidic pH to start with, they will actually help to balance a lot of the foods that are on your meal plan for this coming week, because most fruits and vegetables become alkaline once they have been digested and broken down into other chemical components.

Vegan-Friendly Dietary Fats

There are a wide variety of ingredients vegans and vegetarians can include in their intermittent fasting regimes and still generate higher energy and fat stores.

If you have convictions or dietary restrictions that don't lend themselves to the high fat diets that meats tend to offer, here are five ways to add healthy high fat foods into your diet. And you don't have to be vegetarian or vegan to enjoy them.

1. Avocados

If you are a vegan, you should be stocking avocados in your fridge at all times. They lend themselves to any recipe that requires a creamy base. That very creaminess is a hint that they are high in fats – the healthy monounsaturated kind.

2. Coconut Oil

Unfortunately, clarified butter isn't an option for vegans because it is dairy. If you are vegan, try coconut oil instead. The flavor is fabulous, and it has a high smoking point which means you can deep fry almost anything in it. Coconut oil is a good source of medium-chain triglycerides which can be metabolized in the liver and used directly as an energy source.

3. Cocoa

When I talk about cocoa, I am not talking about hot chocolate and certainly not the candy that comes in wrappers. I am talking about the pure cocoa that comes in melted or powder form. Dark chocolate without the dairy and the sugar is a great source of energy and fat and should be part of your desert options.

4. Seeds

You can add seeds to all kinds of dishes or eat them on the side. They typically pack a large energy punch. Seeds are naturally designed to hold concentrated energy for the new plant until it can start extracting its own from the soil and sun.

One of the most nutritious seeds is the Inca Peanut. You can find them online by searching for "Savi Seed." They have loads of omega-3 and other nutrients. If you want to add them to soups and salads, they provide a good counter balance to spices and herbs. They are as much a super food as chia seeds and sunflower seeds. Consume them with meals during the induction and intermediate week if you can. They will help retrain your appetite for more places to find omega-3 and omega-6.

On the topic of omega-3 and omega-6, it is possible to have too much omega-3. In fact, there is a magic ratio for staying healthy. Ideally, you should have 1 portion of omega-3 to 4-6 parts of omega-6.

5. Nuts

Seeds and nuts are very different things. Seeds are the parts that grow into a new plant. Put them into the ground, water them, and they will sprout. Nuts, on the other hand, have hard shells that reveal the fruit inside when opened. A seed may be still further inside.

Nuts typically contain lots of protein and monounsaturated fats, and are great for vegans and vegetarians who aren't including meat fats and proteins in their diets. For non-vegetarians, nuts can introduce too many carbohydrates. Don't stop eating nuts, but simply be aware of it, and eat less if necessary.

21 Recipes

You can eat anything you want or your heart desires, as long as it is within a certain "window" of time, and it doesn't include processed foods.

Typical intermittent fasting diets don't say anything about the nutritional density of foods, or what you can and cannot eat, but if all you do is to fast intermittently, while continuing to poison your body with chemicals and processed foods, then not only is intermittent fasting going to be harder to do, it's also going to give you fewer results, and, eventually, you will give up.

So, let's just stick to eating healthy. Beyond that, you can eat as much as you feel like eating, and you can eat anything you like, just within specific widows of time while you get used to the process.

ABC Omelet (Apple, Bacon, Cheese)

2 tablespoons clarified butter, melted

3 slices streaky bacon

1 granny smith apple, cubed

2 eggs, whisked

2 oz. (57 g) blue cheese, crumbled

Melt the butter in a skillet and fry the bacon until crispy. Remove the bacon onto a paper towel. Add the cubed apple to the skillet and toss over medium heat. Reduce heat to low and continue cooking until the apple pieces turn golden. When they do, remove, and set aside.

Continue with the same skillet, using the remaining grease from the clarified butter and the bacon, increasing the heat to medium. Add the eggs and blue cheese and cook.

You shouldn't need to add salt – but if you do want to add more salt to taste, wait until the dish is served.

Serve the omelet on a plate, topped with the bacon and apples.

Yield: 1 serving

Aioli Fish

1 fillet white fish

2 tablespoons aioli (see recipe in induction week)

2 tablespoons parmesan cheese, grated

2 tablespoons clarified butter

Preheat oven to 340° F (170° C).

Spread aioli over both sides of the fish. Sprinkle both sides with parmesan.

Grease a baking pan with clarified butter. Place the fillet on the baking pan. Bake for 25 minutes furthest from the heat source.

Yield: 1 serving

Broiled Cod

6 cod fillets

¼ cup olive oil

3 tablespoons white wine vinegar

½ cup clarified butter, melted

1 tablespoon lemon juice

1 tablespoon spicy mustard

1 clove garlic, crushed

sea salt

ground black pepper

1 tablespoon fresh basil, chopped

Preheat the oven to 350° F (175° C).

Put the fish into a Ziplock bag. Add olive oil and vinegar and shake well.

Remove fish from bag and lay out in a baking pan lined with parchment. Bake until cooked through.

Combine clarified butter, lemon juice, mustard, garlic, salt, and pepper in a food processor. Run until smooth.

To serve, pour sauce over the fish, and sprinkle with basil.

Yield: 3 servings

By the Border Omelet

3 eggs

½ red onion, diced

habanero peppers, diced

2 tablespoons clarified butter

Monterey jack cheese, cubed

jalapeño jack cheese, cubed

tabasco sauce

sea salt

ground black pepper

3 tablespoons salsa

Whisk the eggs in a bowl until foamy. Drop in the diced peppers and onions.

Melt clarified butter in a skillet until it starts to sizzle. Tilt the skillet with one hand, allowing the sizzling butter to pool on one side of the tipped skillet. Use your free hand to pour the whisked eggs into the pool of butter. Level and return the skillet to the stove. This technique reduces the possibility of the eggs burning or cooking unevenly.

Sprinkle the cubed cheeses evenly over the eggs. Add salt, pepper, and a few dashes of tobasco sauce to taste.

Serve the cooked omelete warm topped with salsa.

Yield: 1 serving

Denver Omelet

2 tablespoons clarified butter

2 eggs

¼ small onion, sliced

1 oz. (28 g) cheddar cheese, shredded

¼ c. cooked ham, diced

¼ green pepper, sliced

sriracha chili sauce (optional)

Whisk the eggs and onions in a bowl until foamy.

Melt clarified butter in a small skillet until it starts to sizzle. Tilt the skillet with one hand and allow the sizzling butter to pool on one side. Using your free hand, pour the whisked eggs into the butter. Level the skillet and return it to the stove. This technique reduces the possibility of the eggs burning or cooking unevenly.

Sprinkle ham, cheese, and green pepper into the uncooked portion of the eggs. When partially cooked, flip it all over to finish cooking.

Add salt and pepper to taste.

This goes well with sriracha chili sauce if you want some added zing.

Yield: 1 serving

Ceviche

32 oz. (900 g) fresh fish (your choice), filleted

10 green limes (avg. size), juiced, seeds removed

3 green limes (avg. size), juiced separately, seeds removed

4 ripe tomatoes, skinned, seeds and core removed, diced

2 black avocados, skinned, cored, diced

3 fresh jalapeños, skinned, cored, finely diced

½ red onion, skinned, diced

1/3 cup fresh oregano, chopped

1/3 cup fresh cilantro, chopped

sea salt

ground black pepper

For this dish to work, everything must be fresh. Nothing can be frozen and thawed. Once a fish has been frozen and thawed, it affects the texture and taste of this dish.

Cut the fish fillet into bite-sized pieces and put into a crock or another similar container. Pour the juice of the 10 limes over the fish. Gently toss the fish and bath it in the juice until all the fish is fully coated. (There should be enough lime juice that the fish floats freely in it.) Cover and marinate overnight in the fridge for a total of 12 hours. Toss the ingredients frequently before you turn in for the night, and then again when you wake in the morning. This step will cure the raw fish. The fish is "cooked" when all of it has turned white.

Combine tomatoes, jalapenos, avocado, and red onion in a separate bowl.

After marinating the fish, drain the lime juice. Gently remove the fish from the crock or container and add the drained fish to the bowl containing the diced vegetables.

Add cilantro, oregano, salt, and black pepper to the juice of the three remaining limes. Pour this juice mixture onto the fish and vegetables and toss. Serve chilled.

Yield: 3 servings for dinner (or 6 servings as an appetizer)

Cheesy Omelet

2 tablespoons clarified butter

2 eggs

2 oz. (57 g) cheddar cheese, shredded

2 oz. (57 g) monterey jack cheese, shredded

1 oz. (28 g) swiss cheese, chopped

fine sea salt

ground black pepper

lemon wedge

Use an electric whisk to aerate the eggs as you beat them - the more froth and foam, the better. Add a dash of salt to the eggs.

Melt the clarified butter in a small skillet over low heat until it starts to sizzle. Tilt the skillet with one hand and allow the sizzling butter to pool on one side. Use your free hand to pour the whisked eggs into that pool of butter. Level the skillet and return it to the stove. This reduces the possibility of the eggs burning or cooking unevenly.

As the bottom cooks sprinkle the shredded cheeses over the eggs.

Fold the omelet over and cook until a knife stuck in the middle comes out clean.

Slide the omelet out onto a plate to serve. Garnish with salt, pepper, and lemon.

Yield: 1 serving

Cheezy Lamb

½ lb. (228 g) roast lamb, cubed

sea salt

5-8 tbsp. clarified butter

1 onion, chopped

4 tablespoons parmesan cheese

3 tablespoons mayonnaise

2 eggs

Salt lamb and set aside to rest in a colander. The salt will pull out excess moisture from the meat.

Melt 2 tablespoons of the clarified butter in a skillet over medium heat until the butter sizzles. Sauté the lamb cubes till golden brown. Add the onion to the lamb and continue frying until softened. Set aside to cool.

Once cooled, add the lamb and onions to a food processor. Also add the parmesan cheese, mayonnaise, and any butter that remains in the skillet. Run the food processor until thoroughly mixed. Remove mixture from the food processor and set aside.

In a bowl, whisk the eggs and 3 tablespoons of the clarified butter together until foamy.

Melt 2 tablespoons of clarified butter in a skillet until it starts to sizzle. Tilt the skillet with one hand, allowing the melted butter to pool on one side. Use your free hand to pour the eggs into the pool of butter. Level the skillet and return it to the stove. This method reduces the possibility of the eggs burning or cooking unevenly.

Dump the lamb mix into the cooking eggs and fold twice.

Yield: 1 serving

Chinese Steamed Fish

12 oz. (340 g) cod fillet

2 teaspoons fresh ginger, grated

½ teaspoon fresh garlic, minced

1 tablespoon chinese rice wine

1 tablespoon soy sauce

1½ teaspoons toasted sesame oil

2 scallions, minced

You need a deep wok or skillet with a steamer rack that can support a shallow aluminum platter, and a lid to cover everything.

Bring water to a boil in the wok or skillet.

Lightly salt the cod, and sprinkle with grated ginger and garlic. Lay the cod out on the aluminum platter. Place the platter with the cod onto the steamer rack in the wok or skillet. Cover.

Mix rice wine, soy sauce, sesame oil, and scallions in a separate bowl.

Once the cod is fully steamed (the flesh will turn translucent white), remove it from the wok or skillet, and drizzle the soy sauce mixture over it. Serve immediately.

Yield: 2 servings

Cream Baked Sole

1 lb. (454 g) sole fillets

1 cup plain yogurt

½ cup mayonnaise

juice of 1 lemon

paprika

clarified butter

Preheat oven to 330°F (165° C).

Whisk together yogurt, mayonnaise, lemon juice, and paprika. Divide the mixture into two equal portions. One will be used to bake the fish; reserve the other to use as a dip.

Grease a baking dish with clarified butter. Lay soul fillets out in the dish. Spread one portion of the sauce mix over the fillets. Bake in oven for 40 minutes.

Once done, serve with reserved sauce on the side.

Yield: 3 servings

English Muffins

½ cup warm water

½ cup yogurt

1 teaspoon salt

2 ½ oz. (70 g) wheat gluten

¼ cup psyllium husk

2 tablespoons wheat germ

¼ cup wheat bran

½ cup oat flour

½ cup whey powder

2 drops vanilla extract

2 teaspoons yeast

2 tablespoons clarified butter

Combine all ingredients except the clarified butter in a mixer with a dough hook attachment. Once mixed, use a damp cloth to cover the bowl with the dough, and set aside for 30 minutes.

Return bowl to the mixer and run on low setting for 30 seconds. Remove dough and lay out on a clean surface. Flatten and spread the dough out into a ½ in. (1.25 cm) thick square. Using a circular dough cutter, cut out 2-4 circles. Gather the excess dough into a ball, flatten, and cut out more circles. Lay dough circles out on a greased pan, cover with a clean damp cloth, and allow to rise.

Melt clarified butter in a heavy skillet over low heat, thoroughly coating the skillet. Place the risen dough circles neatly into the skillet and cover. Fry until the sides turn brown, then flip them over. Continue cooking until you are confident they are completely cooked through on the inside.

Yield: About 6-7 muffins

Ginger Salmon

1 salmon fillet, skin on

1 clove fresh garlic, crushed

½ inch fresh ginger root, grated

2 tablespoons fresh cilantro, chopped

2 scallions, minced

½ cup white wine

2 tablespoons clarified butter

sea salt

ground black pepper

8 tablespoons sour cream

Combine garlic, ginger, cilantro, scallions, and white wine.

Heat the clarified butter in a heavy skillet and sauté the salmon for 4 minutes on each side. Add the white wine/herb mixture to the skillet. Cook for another 3 minutes. Season to taste with salt and pepper.

To serve, spoon the sauce over the fish, and top with a generous dollop of sour cream.

Yield: 2 servings

Homemade Sour Cream

6 tablespoons buttermilk

2 cups heavy cream

Make the sour cream 2 days ahead of use.

Mix the heavy cream with the buttermilk. Leave in the bottom shelf of the fridge for two days.

Flounder Tarragon & Asparagus

26 oz. (750 g) flounder fillet

30 asparagus spears

sea salt

homemade sour cream (as above)

juice of 1 lemon

Prepare asparagus by snapping woody part off each spear at the base. Bring a pot of salted water to a boil. Drop in the asparagus. Cook for 3 minutes, remove, and blanch in cold running water.

In a separate bowl, mix the homemade sour cream, mustard, and tarragon.

Sprinkle the flounder with sea salt and coat with aioli. Heat a skillet and add two tablespoons of clarified butter and sauté the fish fillet. Once cooked, remove the flounder, leaving excess oil in the skillet.

Place the fish on a serving plate. Drizzle with lemon juice. Place a dollop of the sour cream sauce on the fish. Carefully lay out asparagus on that.

Yield: 2 servings

Pan-Seared Sea Bass

2 lbs. (907 g) sea bass fillets

juice of 1 lemon

2 tablespoon Old Bay Seasoning

8 slices bacon

½ cup clarified butter, melted

Slice the fillets into serving-sized pieces. Gently toss to thoroughly coat the fish in half of the lemon juice. Sprinkle the fish evenly with Old Bay Seasoning.

Use a deep skillet and render the bacon. Remove the bacon, leaving the bacon fat. Fry the sea bass in the sizzling bacon grease for 4 minutes. Flip, and fry for another 4 minutes.

To serve, pour clarified butter over the fish, and sprinkle with remaining lemon juice. Garnish with bacon pieces.

Yield: 6 servings

Pork Frittatas

12 eggs

½ cup parmesan cheese, grated

1 tablespoon lard

½ lb. (225 g) pork sausage, crumbled

½ cup sweet red onion, diced

½ cup green pepper, diced

½ cup sweet red pepper, diced

1 teaspoon fine sea salt

You will need a skillet that can go in the oven and an oven with a broiler.

Beat the eggs in a bowl for 3-4 minutes. Add the parmesan cheese.

Melt the lard in the skillet over medium heat. Add crumbled sausage and brown. When the sausage is light brown, add the onions and continue stirring until the onions soften. Then add green peppers. Sprinkle lightly with salt. Distribute the meat and vegetables evenly in the bottom of the pan. Reduce to low heat.

Pour the beaten eggs over the contents of the skillet. Cover the skillet with an oven-safe lid or aluminum foil and cook for 2 minutes.

Move the covered skillet into the oven, under the broiler, and cook for 10 minutes.

Yield: 6 servings

Rice Bran Bread

9 ½ oz. (270 ml) water

1 oz. (30 g) rice bran

3/4 oz. (20 g) flaxseed meal

3 ½ oz. (100 g) wheat gluten

1 ½ oz. (40 g) whey protein powder

2 teaspoons blackstrap molasses

1 teaspoon sea salt

½ oz. (15 ml) clarified butter

2 teaspoons yeast

A bread maker is required.

Put all ingredients into the bread maker. Set the program for light or dark skin, as desired.

Yield: 10 slices

Sautéed Sole in Balsamic Vinegar

2 lbs. (907 g) sole fillets

white wine vinegar

sea salt

ground black pepper

4 tablespoons clarified butter

½ cup white wine

1 tablespoon fresh oregano

¼ cup balsamic vinegar

2 tablespoon olive oil

1 cup shredded Parmesan cheese

3 lemon wedges

Place the sole fillets in a bowl. Pour in the white wine vinegar and sloshing it around to rinse all the fish. Once the fish has been rinsed in it, discard the vinegar, and lay the fish out on paper towels to dry.

Sprinkle the fish with salt and pepper. Gently rub the seasoning into both sides of the fish with your hands.

Melt butter in a skillet and heat until sizzling. Sauté the fillets on both sides. Use a slotted spoon and a wooden spatula to hold the fillets carefully as you turn them over.

Pour the white wine into the skillet, without pouring it on the fish. Let the wine slowly sizzle, allowing the alcohol to evaporate. Sprinkle the oregano over the fish. Continue cooking until the wine fully evaporates.

Remove the sole from the skillet and lay out on a plate. Add the balsamic vinegar, drizzle with olive oil, and sprinkle with parmesan cheese. Serve with a wedge of lemon on the side.

Yield: 3 servings

Sea Bass in Heavy Cream

12 oz. (340 g) sea bass filleted

3 tablespoons olive oil

½ lb. (225 g) mixed olives, pitted, washed

2 anchovy fillets, sliced

2 tablespoons capers

2 fresh basil leaves, crushed

juice of 1 lemon

2 tablespoons extra virgin olive oil

2 tablespoons clarified butter

¼ onion, sliced thinly

2 cloves garlic, crushed

1 tablespoon balsamic vinegar

3 tablespoons heavy cream

sea salt

ground black pepper

Pre-heat broiler. Divide sea bass fillets into two portions. Brush 3 tablespoons of olive oil on all sides. Broil the fish as you prepare the sauce.

To make tapenade, combine the olives, anchovies, capers, basil, lemon juice, and the 2 tablespoons extra virgin olive oil in a food processor. Run until you get a smooth paste. Set aside.

Sauté onions and garlic with the 2 tablespoons of butter in a heavy skillet for 5 minutes. Add the tapenade and balsamic vinegar to the skillet. Continue sautéing for 2 minutes. Remove from heat and let rest for 2 minutes. Stir in the cream.

Spoon the sauce over the fish to serve. Add salt and pepper to taste.

Yield: 2 servings

Spanish Tilapia

4 whole tilapias filleted

¾ teaspoon paprika

juice of 3 limes

2 tablespoons clarified butter

½ cup clarified butter

1 medium red onion, thinly sliced

¼ teaspoon ground cumin

3 tablespoons orange juice

½ teaspoon habanero sauce

1 tablespoon white wine vinegar

1 tablespoon fresh oregano

sea salt

ground black pepper

Arrange the tilapia fillets on a flat plate. Mix 1/3 of the lime juice in a separate bowl with the paprika. Drench both sides of the fish with the juice mixture.

Melt 2 tablespoons butter in a heavy skillet and sauté fillets until golden on each side. Remove fish and place in an oven-safe serving dish. Keep dish warm in the oven. Leave the grease in the skillet.

Add the ½ cup of clarified butter to the skillet, melting it over medium heat. When it sizzles, add the onions, and sauté until soft and brown. Add cumin, stirring until fragrant. Add remaining lime juice, orange juice, habanero sauce, white wine vinegar, and oregano. Stir over medium-low heat for about 2 minutes.

To serve, spoon the onion sauce over the tilapia.

Yield: 4 servings

Tilapia with Vegetables

1 lb. (454 g) tilapia fillets

sea salt

white pepper

3 tablespoons clarified butter

2 cups red pepper, sliced

2 cups yellow pepper, sliced

2 cups zucchini, sliced

2 cups squash, diced

2 cups red onion, diced

1 clove garlic, crushed

¾ tablespoon corn flour

lemon wedges

Rub the sea salt and white pepper onto the tilapia fillets and set aside.

Melt the butter in a skillet. Sauté the vegetables, onions, and garlic for 4 to 5 minutes, stirring frequently. Lay the fish over the vegetables in the skillet, and cover. Keep heat at medium. Cook for 10 minutes in the steam.

Lay out the fish out on a serving dish and shimmy the vegetables onto the fish, retaining the liquids in the skillet. Return the skillet to the heat, and when the sauce is sizzling, add in the corn flour, continuing to stir until the sauce thickens. Pour the thickened sauce over the vegetables and fish. Serve with lemon wedges.

Yield: 4 servings

Chapter 5: Advanced "Booster" Week

Advanced "Booster" Week is all about boosting the way your body asks for food. By getting your metabolism to switch tracks for longer periods of time, you can be a continuous fat-burning machine rather than a fat-storing machine.

"Booster" Schedule

This schedule is fairly easy to follow. It is organized according to "windows" of time. During 2-hour meal windows, you have full meals – full meals are defined as whatever you want to eat and however much you can eat without feeling over-full. The key is to always listen to your body. These are alternated with fasting no-meal windows. During those periods of fasting, remember to keep drinking the lemon water, and stay hydrated.

Meal	DAY						
	1	2	3	4	5	6	7
7am - 9am	0	MD2	0	0	MD5	0	0
11am - 1pm	0	0	0	0	0	0	0
6pm - 8pm	ED1	0	0	ED4	0	0	ED7

The basic schedule follows a 7:2 pattern. Two meal windows follow each other, ED1 and MD2, for instance. These are followed by seven windows of no meals. That is followed by two meal time windows and another seven fasting windows. This 7:2 formula is designed to alter the metabolism, activating the body's fat-burning metabolism for longer periods. The foods in the booster week recipes below will also help with that goal.

Chicken Pie

2 lbs. (907 g) chicken (dark, no skin), chopped

1 quart (1.1 L) chicken broth

2 tablespoons clarified butter

1 cup baking flour

¼ lb. (115 g) carrots, diced

¼ lb. (115 g) peas

¼ lb. (115 g) green beans, cut in ½ inch pieces

1 cup shitake mushrooms, sliced

1 cup almond milk

sea salt

ground black pepper

corn flour

Put chopped chicken and broth into a pressure cooker. Pressurize and cook for 30 minutes.

Once the chicken is done, release the pressure and open the cover. Remove the chicken pieces and drain in a colander. Remove and strain one cup of broth, leaving the remaining broth in the pot.

Combine the strained cup of broth, baking flour, and clarified butter in a mixing bowl. Knead until it forms a soft dough, then fold it over on itself numerous times.

Flour a flat surface and lay the dough on it. Use a rolling pin to flatten the dough. Fold it again, then roll it. Repeat five times. The dough should be ¼ inch thick.

Line the inside of an oven-safe glass bowl with the flattened dough, letting the excess hang over the sides. Set aside.

Add the vegetables (carrots, peas, green beans, and mushrooms) to the hot broth in the pot. Cook for about 4-5 minutes. Add the almond milk. Add corn flour to the broth and keep stirring until it thickens. Season with salt and pepper.

Return the chicken to the pot with the thickened broth and veggies. Mix thoroughly.

Scoop the chicken, vegetables, and gravy into the dough-lined bowl. Fold the excess dough back on top of it.

Bake in the oven for 20 minutes.

Serve warm, using a large serving spoon to scoop out the crust and chicken mixture.

Yield: 6 servings

Dumplings

1 quart (1.1 L) chicken broth

1 cup ground almonds

½ cup rice protein powder

¼ cup wheat flour

2 tablespoons clarified butter

2 tablespoons coconut oil

½ teaspoon fine sea salt

2 teaspoons baking powder

½ teaspoon baking soda

¾ cup plain yogurt

Set the chicken broth to boil in a pot.

Pulse all remaining ingredients, except the yogurt, in a food processor until fully mixed. Add the yogurt and fold everything together. You should now have a soft dough.

Using a spoon, scoop half-tablespoons of the dough and drop into the boiling broth. Cook over medium-high heat for 30 minutes.

Yield: 12 servings

Egg Drop Soup

1 quart (1.1 L) chicken broth

1 tablespoon coconut aminos (soy sauce replacement)

1 tablespoon umeboshi vinegar (ume plum vinegar)

½ teaspoon fresh ginger, grated

1 scallion, finely sliced

2 eggs

ground white pepper

Heat the broth in a saucepan over medium-high heat. Add coconut amino, umeboshi vinegar, ginger, and scallion. Simmer for 4 minutes.

Beat the eggs lightly in a bowl.

Once the broth is boiling, pour the beaten egg into the broth, slowly as one continuous stream . Don't pour the egg all at once or drip it in. Pour the egg in one long, controlled stream, while stirring the broth in a circular motion.

Serve with pepper to taste.

Yield: 4 Servings

Ground Beef Stir-Fry

1 lb. (454 g) ground beef

2 tablespoons coconut aminos

3 tablespoons chinese cooking wine

2 cloves garlic, crushed

sea salt

3 tablespoons (or more) coconut oil

½ cup peanuts, coarsely chopped

1½ teaspoons fresh ginger, grated

1 cup green beans, chopped

1 cup broccoli, chopped

1 medium onion, sliced

1 teaspoon fish sauce

Combine 1 tablespoon of the coconut aminos, 1 tablespoon of the cooking wine, a pinch of sea salt and the garlic. Massage that into the ground beef. Separate the ground beef mix into bite-sized chunks.

Heat 3 tablespoons coconut oil in a deep wok over high heat. Fry the peanuts until golden. Remove and set aside.

Fry the ground beef chunks in the oil after removing the peanuts. Remove the beef.

Add more oil if necessary and sauté the ginger until fragrant. Remove and set aside.

Fry the green beans, broccoli, and onion for 2-4 minutes until cooked. Return the beef, peanuts, and ginger to the wok. Toss everything together, adding the fish sauce, remaining coconut aminos, and remaining cooking wine.

Yield: 3 servings

Lemon-Glazed Turkey Cutlets

3 turkey breasts, cubed

rosemary, finely chopped

1 tablespoon clarified butter

1 tablespoon lemon juice

½ teaspoon coconut aminos

3 scallions, thinly sliced

sea salt

ground black pepper

Pulse turkey, rosemary, and salt in a food processor until the meat is chunky. Form the mixture into patties by hand.

Heat clarified butter in a heavy skillet until sizzling. Fry the turkey patties until brown. Remove and set aside.

Combine lemon juice, coconut aminos, scallions, salt, and pepper. Heat this lemon juice mixture in the skillet. Pour this glaze over the turkey patties before serving.

Yield: 2 or 3 servings

Mushroom Turkey Wings

4 lbs. (1.8 Kg) turkey wings

1 cup clarified butter

½ medium onion, sliced

1 cup mushrooms, sliced

1 tablespoon tomato paste

½ cup chicken broth

sea salt

1 tablespoon corn flour

½ cup sour cream

Melt butter in a cast iron dutch oven over high heat until sizzling. Pan fry the turkey wings until brown. Add onions and fry until brown. Add the mushrooms. Cover and cook for 10 minutes.

Stir in the tomato paste. Add the chicken broth. Season with sea salt. Cover and boil for 10 minutes.

Remove turkey wings and set aside.

Stir corn flour into the pan to thicken the broth. Add sour cream and stir.

Serve the turkey wings with the sauce.

Yield: 3 servings

Mustard Turkey Cutlets

3 turkey breast cutlets or turkey breasts

½ cup raw almonds

1 tablespoon chinese hot mustard

3 tablespoons eggless mayonnaise

3 tablespoons clarified butter

Brown almonds in a dry frypan. Use a food processor to chop the almonds until fine. Add the mustard and eggless mayonnaise and continue blending.

Coat the turkey with the almond mix.

Melt butter in a heavy skillet until sizzling. Fry turkey until browned.

To serve, pour the grease from the pan and any almond scrapings over the turkey.

Yield: 2 Servings

Prosciutto Salad

14 oz. (400 g) artichoke hearts, cut in bite-sized pieces

3.5 oz. (100 g) prosciutto, thinly sliced, cut into 1 x ¼ inch pieces (25 x 6 mm)

½ cup pitted olives, chopped

1 large tomato, skinned and diced

¼ cup fresh basil, finely chopped

3 tablespoons extra virgin olive oil

4 teaspoons white wine vinegar

2 cloves garlic, crushed

½ teaspoon spicy mustard

Combine artichoke hearts, prosciutto strips, olive pieces, diced tomato, and basil in a bowl. Toss together.

Combine olive oil, vinegar, garlic, and mustard. Add this dressing to the bowl and toss all together thoroughly.

Let sit for 20 minutes in the fridge before serving.

Yield: 4 servings

Stracciatella

1 tablespoon bacon grease

1 fresh rosemary sprig, finely chopped

½ teaspoon fresh nutmeg, grated

1 quart (1.1 L) chicken broth

2 eggs, lightly beaten

1 tablespoon balsamic vinegar

1 tablespoon lemon juice

ground black pepper to taste

½ cup grated parmesan cheese

Heat bacon grease in pot. Sauté rosemary and nutmeg. Add chicken broth and bring to boil. Pour beaten eggs into the boiling soup while stirring. When the eggs are firm, add vinegar, lemon juice, and pepper.

Distribute broth to serving sized oven-safe bowls. Top with parmesan cheese. Place under broiler until the cheese melts. Serve warm.

Yield: 4 servings

Submarine Salad

8 cups rocket lettuce

½ lb. (227 g) prosciutto

¼ lb. (113 g) mortadella

¼ lb. (113 g) salami

¼ lb. (113 g) smoked provolone cheese, sliced

¼ lb. (113 g) mozzarella cheese, sliced

1 red onion, sliced

3 tablespoons roasted red pepper, chopped

4 fresh basil leaves, chopped

1 large tomato, skinned, cored and sliced

2 tablespoons extra virgin olive oil

1 clove garlic, crushed

1 tablespoon red wine vinegar

pinch ground black pepper

pinch sea salt

Make a bed of rocket lettuce on a large serving plate.

Slice all the cheese and meats into strips 1 inch (2.5 cm) long by ¼ inch (.6 cm) wide.

On the bed of lettuce, layer a little cheese, then a little meat, then a little cheese again, alternating the sliced ingredients.

Just before serving, top with the onions, red pepper, basil, and tomato.

Blend olive oil, garlic, wine vinegar, black pepper, and salt to make a dressing. Pour this dressing over all the ingredients on the serving platter.

Yield: 2 servings

A Healthy Intermittent Fasting Lifestyle

Having reached the end of three weeks of intermittent fasting, you are now truly a new person, functioning in a different way, restoring your mind and body to a way of consuming food that is more in line with that of our ancestors of 50,000 years ago. These three weeks of discipline have been designed to change the body in such a way that it has stopped responding to food in habitual ways and has therefore stopped being derailed by those habits. The idea has been to get your body to make the right choices regardless of what the mind is saying.

During the past three weeks, you have also been scrubbed of the toxins usually contained in processed foods, allowing you to be truer to your natural appetites. You won't just crave flavorful or pleasing foods that have empty calories but you will have an appetite for the things your body really needs.

Shifting how your body asks for food is an important element in eating healthy, but we went one step further. Not only did we start getting your body to ask for the right food, we got your body to ask for it at the right time, when it needed it. We changed the basic philosophy of eating: now we look to stored food to energize us instead of eating to increase stores.

We also looked to expand the range of food choices, rather than restricting it. Fasts that cut out what you eat and reduce it to certain areas are not healthy because they reduce the diversity of your choices. Our body needs hundreds of different compounds (enzymes, vitamins, minerals, proteins, and more), so we cannot just limit our diet to a few food sources. The more you diversify your foods, the more your body will get what it needs, and will add to its "library" of sources for what it needs.

The "what" and "when" of eating is what intermittent fasting is all about. The "when" is easy to discern – we eat when our body needs it. The "what" is anything we want to eat – as long as it isn't processed or something that harms us.

Now, having gotten this far, you should stop looking at the eating schedules as rigid plans and begin to see them as guardrails. That means you should eat what you feel like and only when you feel hungry. If you find you are eating too often and/or too much, and the weight is creeping back on, then you can pull back. Otherwise, leave the timing of meals, the amount to eat, and the items to eat to the dictates of your own body. Remember, weight loss can occur naturally in intermittent fasting because stored fat is being used as fuel.

Not only do you have access to a higher quality source of energy when you do this, you also allow the body more time to clean up, get healthy, and get alert. Remember when we talked about the protein shells – those "bags" that carry fats to their destinations? The body needs time to clean that up. Fasting perfectly provides time for your body to digest and flush all those protein packets out of your system after they have been used. That is the reason my LDL levels dropped after my first 30-day fast. Intermittent fasting gives your body time to make repairs to all its issues.

I especially want to remind you to drink plenty of water. You don't have to add lemon to your water anymore if you don't want to. The lemon was added mostly to shift your intake toward the alkaline side of the equation because most processed foods are notorious acidifying foods. Switching to a more alkaline diet should have helped to readjust your taste buds.

You should also continue to stay away from sugar – and that really does include sugar substitutes like stevia and all those aspartame derivatives. It is not so much that they are bad for you as that they encourage the habit of wanting sweetness. Learn to take foods as they are without adding the taste of sweet. That sweetness is the lazy way out in terms of energy generation. Sugars give you a quick boost of energy but are never enough to keep you going for long. Triglycerides are a better source of energy and you can get that everywhere because your body makes them from almost everything you eat. Eating healthy foods starts by skewing your taste preferences and cravings toward what is healthy.

Final Thoughts

This brings us to the end of this book on intermittent fasting. I hope it has been of help to you and that you have found the inspiration to experience a new way of eating that will elevate your body's ability to meet its full potential. Intermittent fasting will change the way you move, the way you think, and the way you succeed in all the things that you do.

Happy living!

If you enjoyed learning about Intermittent Fasting I would be forever grateful if you could leave a review on Amazon. Reviews are by far the best way to help your fellow readers find the good books so make sure to help them out!

Appendix: List of Acidic Foods PH

The following is a list of foods with their corresponding pH values. Acidic foods have a pH between 1 and 6.9 – the lower the number the more acidic. Neutral is a pH of 7. Alkaline is from 7.1 to 14. The higher the number, the higher the alkalinity.

Most of the items in this list are fruits and vegetables. Most fruits and vegetables become alkaline in the body after they have been digested, even though they start out as acidic.

Item	Approximate pH
Lemons / Lemon Juice	2.0
Limes / Lime Juice	2.0
Cranberry Juice, canned	2.3
Grenadine Syrup	2.3
Vinegar	2.4
Gelatin Dessert	2.6

Loganberries	2.7
Chili Sauce, acidified	2.8
Gooseberries	2.8
Grapes, Concord	2.8
Grapes, Niagara	2.8
Plums, Blue	2.8
Raspberry Jam	2.9
Grapes, Seedless	2.9
Grapefruit Juice, canned	2.9
Plums, Damson	2.9
Crabapple Jelly	2.9
Pomegranate	2.9
Grapefruit	3.0
Fruit Jellies	3.0
Orange Marmalade	3.0
Strawberries	3.0
Strawberry Jam	3.0
Tamarind	3.0

Youngberries, frozen	3.0
Mint Jelly	3.0
Grapefruit, canned	3.1
Applesauce	3.1
Red Pepper Relish	3.1
Rhubarb	3.1
Cider Vinegar	3.1
Blueberries	3.1
Quince, fresh, stewed	3.1
Raspberries, fresh or frozen	3.2
Apple, baked with sugar	3.2
Cucumbers / Dill Pickles	3.2
Grapes, Muscatine	3.2
Pineapple	3.2
Rhubarb, California, stewed	3.2
Strawberries, frozen	3.2
Plums, frozen	3.2
Plums, Green Gage, canned	3.2

Cherries, red, water packed	3.3
Mayhaw	3.3
Peaches, frozen	3.3
Apricots	3.3
Apricots, dried, stewed	3.3
Orange Juice, California	3.3
Orange Juice, Florida	3.3
Peaches	3.3
Pineapple Juice, canned	3.3
Sauerkraut	3.3
Cherries, frozen	3.3
Strawberries, California	3.3
Tangerine	3.3
Apples, Jonathan	3.3
Apples, McIntosh	3.3
Apple Juice	3.4
Pineapple, canned	3.4
Guava, canned	3.4

Sherry Wine	3.4
Huckleberries, cooked with sugar	3.4
Apricots, canned	3.4
Mangoes, ripe	3.4
Rhubarb, canned	3.4
Apricots, pureed	3.4
Plum Nectar	3.5
Apples, Winesap	3.5
Cherries, Maraschino	3.5
Bamboo Shoots, preserved	3.5
Grapes, canned	3.5
Grapes, Tokyo	3.5
Fruit Jam	3.5
Pears, Bartlett	3.5
Raspberries, New Jersey	3.5
Tomatoes, canned	3.5
Tomato Paste	3.5
Grapes, Lady Finger	3.5

Papaya Marmalade	3.5
Mustard	3.6
Peaches, cooked with sugar	3.6
Apples, Golden Delicious	3.6
Fruit Cocktail	3.6
Olives, green, fermented	3.6
Oranges, Florida, "color added"	3.6
Plums, Green Gage	3.6
Plums, Red	3.6
Prunes, pureed	3.6
Prunes, dried, stewed	3.6
Worcestershire Sauce	3.6
Kumquat, Florida	3.6
Oranges, Florida	3.7
Raspberry Sherbet	3.7
Grapes, Ribier	3.7
Honey	3.7
Onions, pickled	3.7

Peaches, canned	3.7
Quince Jelly	3.7
Grapes, Malaga	3.7
Apricots, strained	3.7
Guava Jelly	3.7
Apricot Nectar	3.8
Cherries, Royal Ann	3.8
Coconut Preserves	3.8
Raisins, seedless	3.8
Cherries, Black, canned	3.8
Tomatillos	3.8
Blackberries, Washington	3.9
Ketchup	3.9
Apples, Delicious	3.9
Plums, Yellow	3.9
Vegetable Juice	3.9
Nectarines	3.9
Prune Juice	4.0

Pears, canned	4.0
Cherries, California	4.0
Pear Nectar	4.0
Pears, Sickle, cooked w/sugar	4.0
Acidophilus Milk	4.1
Cream Cheese, Philadelphia	4.1
Tomato Juice	4.1
Dates, Dromedary	4.1
Cucumbers, pickled	4.2
Artichokes, canned, acidified	4.3
Beets, canned, acidified	4.3
Tomatoes	4.3
Enchilada sauce	4.4
Pimiento/Pimento	4.4
Soy Sauce	4.4
Buttermilk	4.4
Persimmons	4.4
Tomatoes, vine ripened	4.4

Bananas	4.5
Pickled Herring	4.5
Mangosteen	4.5
Taro syrup	4.5
Carrots, pureed	4.6
Bananas, red	4.6
Curry Paste, acidified	4.6
Maple Syrup, light (acidified)	4.6
Cream of Tomato Soup, canned	4.6
Peppers	4.7
Cactus	4.7
Honey Aloe	4.7
Lychee	4.7
Sour Milk, fine curd	4.7
Cottage Cheese	4.8
Asparagus	4.8
Jackfruit	4.8
Zwiebach	4.8

Basil Pesto	4.9
Beets, canned	4.9
Corn Flakes	4.9
Molasses	4.9
Peas, pureed	4.9
Pumpkin	4.9
Rambutan (Thailand)	4.9
Straw Mushroom	4.9
Figs, canned	4.9
Fish Sauce	4.9
Cheese, American, mild	5.0
Vegetable Soup	5.0
Wheat Krispies	5.0
Abalone Mushrooms	5.0
Asparagus, canned	5.0
Banana, yellow	5.0
White Bread	5.0
Nata De Coco	5.0

Oyster Mushrooms	5.0
Satay Sauce	5.0
Shrimp Paste	5.0
Wheaties	5.0
Boston Style Beans	5.1
Figs, Calamyrna	5.1
Mixed Greens, chopped	5.1
Melba Toast	5.1
Bamboo Shoots	5.1
Pork & Beans with Tomato Sauce, canned	5.1
Carrots, strained	5.1
Cheese, Roquefort	5.1
Loquat (may be acidified to pH 3.8)	5.1
Macaroni, cooked	5.1
Potatoes, mashed	5.1
Cucumbers	5.1
Maple syrup	5.2

Vegetable Soup, canned	5.2
Carrots, canned	5.2
Cheese, Snippy	5.2
Acorn Squash, cooked	5.2
Watermelon	5.2
Barley, cooked	5.2
Asparagus, green, canned	5.2
Baby Corn	5.2
Rye Bread	5.2
Broccoli, canned	5.2
Cabbage	5.2
Cheese, Parmesan	5.2
Chives	5.2
Jujube	5.2
Papaya	5.2
Green Peppers	5.2
Rattan, Thailand	5.2
Mixed Greens, strained	5.2

Beets, cooked	5.2
Puffed Wheat	5.3
Turnips	5.3
Wax Beans	5.3
Beets	5.3
Carrots, chopped	5.3
Codfish, boiled	5.3
Milkfish	5.3
Parsnip	5.3
Shallots, cooked	5.3
Sweet Potatoes	5.3
Truffle	5.3
Beans with Tomato Sauce, canned	5.32
Beets, chopped or strained	5.3
Onions, yellow or red	5.3
Wheat Chex	5.3
Breadfruit, cooked	5.3
Horseradish, freshly ground	5.4

Salmon, fresh, broiled	5.4
Celery, cooked	5.4
Onions, white	5.4
Spinach, chopped	5.4
Kidney Beans	5.4
Pumpernickel Bread	5.4
Cheese, Edam	5.4
Potatoes	5.4
Rice Krispies	5.4
Three Bean Salad	5.4
Turnip Greens, cooked	5.4
Sardine, Portuguese, in olive oil	5.4
Walnuts, English	5.4
Cracked Wheat Bread	5.4
Bran Flakes	5.5
Parsnips, cooked	5.5
White Bread Rolls	5.5
Whole Wheat Bread	5.5

Fennel (Anise)	5.5
Leeks, cooked	5.5
Ackees	5.5
Artichokes	5.5
Cabbage, Green	5.5
Coconut, fresh	5.5
Eggplant	5.5
Guava Nectar	5.5
Leeks	5.5
Okra, cooked	5.5
Red Ginseng	5.5
Enchilada Sauce	5.5
Spinach	5.5
Spinach, pureed	5.5
Yams, cooked	5.5
Cream of Coconut, canned	5.5
Radishes, white	5.5
Squash, white, cooked	5.5

Turnip, yellow, cooked	5.6
Carrots, cooked	5.6
Antipasto	5.6
Artichokes, French, cooked	5.6
Beans	5.6
Beans, String	5.6
Cabbage, Red	5.6
Cauliflower	5.6
Four Bean Salad	5.6
Ginger	5.6
Spinach, strained	5.6
Soda Crackers	5.7
Yeast	5.7
Cheese, Swiss Gruyere	5.7
Oysters	5.7
Zucchini, cooked	5.7
Caviar, American	5.7
Celery	5.7

Cheese, Stilton	5.7
Escarole	5.7
Hearts of Palm	5.7
Lettuce, Iceberg	5.7
Lobster Soup	5.7
Matzos	5.7
Parsley	5.7
Peas, canned	5.7
Cream of Pea Soup, canned	5.7
Pork & Beans	5.7
Sardines	5.7
Shad Roe, sauteed	5.7
Celery Knob, cooked	5.7
Kippered Herring, Marshall	5.8
Turnip, white, cooked	5.8
Beans, Black	5.8
Melon, Casaba	5.8
Romaine Lettuce	5.8

Squash, yellow, cooked	5.8
Calamari (Squid)	5.8
Cheese Dip	5.8
Fennel, cooked	5.8
Garlic	5.8
Grass Jelly	5.8
Lentil Soup	5.8
Lettuce	5.8
Mangoes, green	5.8
Vermicelli, cooked	5.8
Radishes, red	5.9
Salmon, fresh, boiled	5.9
Wheatena	5.9
Carrots	5.9
Watercress	5.9
Lettuce, Boston	5.9
Beans, refried	5.9
Cheese, Cheddar	5.9

Chicory	5.9
Corn	5.9
Corn, canned	5.9
Mackerel, canned	5.9
Melons, Persian	5.9
Milk, evaporated	5.9
Pate	5.9
Potato Soup	5.9
Tuna Fish, canned	5.9
Peas, strained	5.9
Scotch Broth	5.9
Artichokes, Jerusalem, cooked	5.9
Baby Food Soup, unstrained	6.0
Cream of Mushroom Soup, canned	5.95
Spaghetti, cooked	6.0
Aloe Juice	6.0
Asparagus	6.0
Soybeans	6.0

Brussels Sprouts	6.0
Capers	6.0
Carp	6.0
Chayote (Mirliton), cooked	6.0
Clams	6.0
Cream of Potato Soup	6.0
Curry sauce	6.0
Korean Ginseng Drink	6.0
Hominy, cooked	6.0
Melons, Honeydew	6.0
Mushrooms	6.0
Mussels	6.0
Octopus	6.0
Olives, black	6.0
Olives, ripe	6.0
Oysters, smoked	6.0
Razor shell (sea asparagus)	6.0
Rice, White, cooked	6.0

Rice, Wild, cooked	6.0
Scallop	6.0
Sea Snail (Top shell)	6.0
Squash, Hubbard, cooked	6.0
Squid	6.0
Water Chestnut	6.0
Asparagus, cooked	6.0
Shredded Wheat	6.1
Cream of Wheat, cooked	6.1
Mackerel, Spanish, broiled	6.1
Salmon, Red Alaska, canned	6.1
Gelatin, plain	6.1
Noodles, boiled	6.1
Bluefish, Boston, broiled	6.1
Abalone	6.1
Aloe Vera	6.1
Asparagus Stalks	6.1
Coconut milk	6.1

Cream of Asparagus	6.1
Egg Yolk	6.1
Flounder, boiled	6.1
Herring	6.1
Cantaloupe	6.1
Cheese, Old English	6.2
Haddock, Filet, broiled	6.2
Swiss Chard, cooked	6.2
Cabbage, White	6.2
Cod Liver	6.2
Dates, canned	6.2
Eel	6.2
Oatmeal, cooked	6.2
Razor Clams	6.2
Rice, Brown, cooked	6.2
Scallion	6.2
Sturgeon	6.2
Trout, Sea, sautéed	6.2

Corn, cooked on cob	6.2
Peas, cooked	6.2
Mackerel, King, boiled	6.3
Avocados	6.3
Puffed Rice	6.3
Peanut Butter	6.3
Broccoli, cooked	6.3
Broccoli, frozen, cooked	6.3
Cabbage, Savoy	6.3
Cuttlefish	6.3
Kelp	6.3
Lentils, cooked	6.3
Spinach, frozen, cooked	6.3
Milk, condensed	6.3
Asparagus, frozen, cooked	6.4
Kale, cooked	6.4
Arrowroot Cruel	6.4
Flounder, fillet, broiled	6.4

Clam Chowder, New England	6.4
Congee	6.4
Milk, cow	6.4
Peas, frozen, cooked	6.4
Porgy, broiled	6.4
Peas, dried (split yellow), cooked	6.43
Cereal, strained	6.4
Cream, 40 per cent	6.4
Cauliflower, cooked	6.5
Peas, dried (split green), cooked	6.45
Milk, goat	6.5
Chick Peas / Garbanzo Beans	6.5
Anchovies	6.5
Striped Bass, broiled	6.5
Beans, Lima	6.5
Crab Meat	6.5
Cream, 20%	6.5
Chrysanthemum Drink	6.5

Shrimp	6.5
Bread, Boston, brown	6.5
Sea Bass, broiled	6.6
Eggs, new-laid, whole	6.6
Soy Infant Formula	6.6
Spinach, cooked	6.6
Crabmeat, cooked	6.6
Arrowroot Crackers	6.6
Smelts, sautéed	6.7
Asparagus Buds	6.7
Hearts of Palm	6.7
Pollack, fillet, broiled	6.7
Lobster Bisque	6.9
Lotus Root	6.9
Soybean Milk	7.0
Shrimp Sauce	7.0
Graham Crackers	7.1
Lobster, cooked	7.1

Milk, peptonized	7.1
Bird's Nest Soup	7.2
Tea	7.2
Tofu (Soybean Curd)	7.2
Wax Gourd Drink	7.2
Corn, frozen	7.3
Cheese, Camembert	7.4
Peanut Soup	7.5
Conch	7.5
Egg White	8.0

Made in the
USA
Monee, IL